Raw*licious*

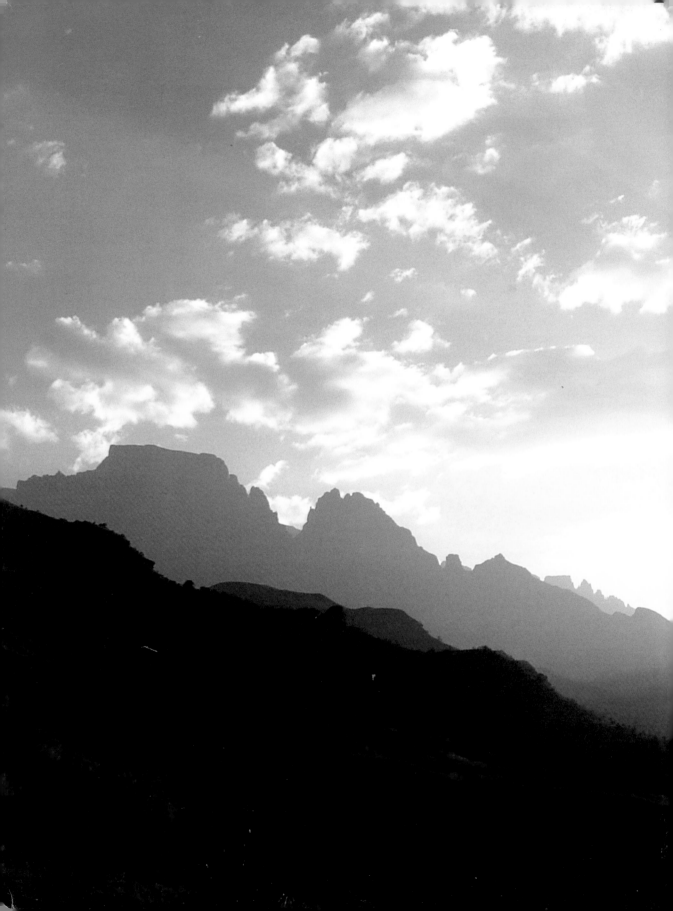

Rawlicious outlines the first few steps across a bridge into a new paradigm. In this magical world we are aware of ourselves as particles within the body of the Earth. In this world we are awake, connected, open, and blissful, and our footsteps are simply whispers in the sand. We look up at the sun and stars, we watch the moon rise over the dark sea and cast its glittering light over the water, we feel the Earth beneath our feet, and marvel with awe and wonder at this vast and expansive dream.

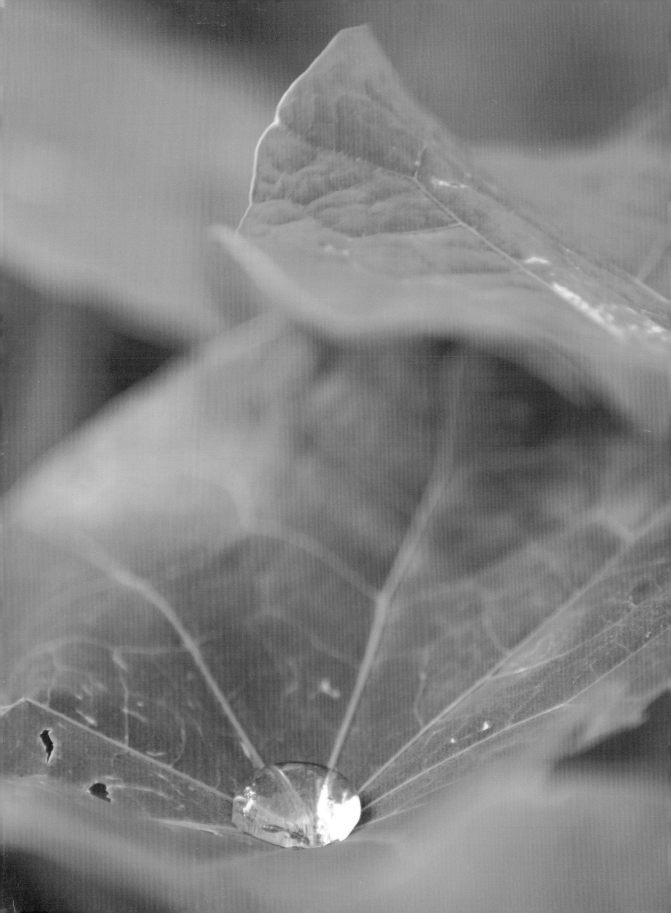

Rawlicious

Delicious Raw Recipes for Radiant Health

PETER AND BERYN DANIEL

Foreword by

VICTORIA BOUTENKO

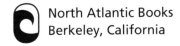

North Atlantic Books
Berkeley, California

Published by
North Atlantic Books
P.O. Box 12327
Berkeley, California 94712

Cover cabbage photo: ©iStockphoto.com/ Sergii Tsololo
Cover food photographs by Allan M Photography
Interior photographs by Allan M Photography, Peter Daniel, and Luke Daniel
Cover design by Paula Morrison
Interior design by Marissa Cuenoud
Printed in the United States of America

Rawlicious: Delicious Raw Recipes for Radiant Health is sponsored by the Society for the Study of Native Arts and Sciences, a nonprofit educational corporation whose goals are to develop an educational and cross-cultural perspective linking various scientific, social, and artistic fields; to nurture a holistic view of arts, sciences, humanities, and healing; and to publish and distribute literature on the relationship of mind, body, and nature.

MEDICAL DISCLAIMER: The following information is intended for general information purposes only. Individuals should always see their health care provider before administering any suggestions made in this book. Any application of the material set forth in the following pages is at the reader's discretion and is his or her sole responsibility.

North Atlantic Books' publications are available through most bookstores. For further information, visit our Web site at www.northatlanticbooks.com or call 800-733-3000.

Library of Congress Cataloging-in-Publication Data
Daniel, Peter, 1980–
  Rawlicious : delicious raw recipes for radiant health / Peter and Beryn Daniel.
       p. cm.
  Originally published: Cape Town, South Africa : Soaring Free Superfoods, 2009.
  Summary: "Two traditionally trained chefs turned raw have created this inviting guide to raw food living and cuisine with a flair for beauty, taste, and presentation"—Provided by publisher.
  ISBN 978-1-55643-965-0 (pbk.)
  1. Vegetarian cooking. 2. Raw food diet. 3. Raw foods. 4. Cookbooks. I. Daniel, Beryn, 1979– II. Title.
  TX837.D2214 2011
  641.5′636—dc22
                          2010049124

1 2 3 4 5 6 7 8 9 United 16 15 14 13 12 11

This book could not have come together without the intricate weaving of the hand of the Spirit. When things are meant to be, they flow, and this book is an expression of that flow. The right people have appeared at the right time to offer not only their skills but their laughter and enthusiasm, too. Without them you would be looking at blank pages.

Firstly, we have to thank each and every one of you who have attended our raw food events and asked, "When are you going to write a book?" It is your desire to see these recipes compiled in a book that gave birth to this project.

THANKS

To Mom, for wholeheartedly supporting our vision from the start.
To Mom and Dad, for your constant encouragement, valuable advice, and for providing us with a quiet haven by the sea to work on this book uninterrupted.
To Barbara, for being an inspirational elder and for seeing our potential when we were just sprouts.
To Lexi, not just for all the hours spent with us in the kitchen, but for turning late nights of recipe trials into kitchen jols.
To Marissa, for artistically bringing this book to life with the style, flair, and efficiency that is inherently you.
To Allan, for vibing with us in the kitchen and taking such delectable photographs.
To Luke, for snapping away and capturing our pasta-making day on camera.
To Gayleen, Callan, Eunice, and Stan for keeping the Soaring Free Superfoods office running smoothly and efficiently so we could focus on this book.
To Anthea, for graciously and generously letting us take over your beautiful kitchen.
To Soil for Life, for lending us your abundant garden for a day.
To the Ethical Co-op and Organic Zone, for keeping us in constant supply of gorgeous, fresh, organic produce.
To Rob, Kirsty, Callan, Werner and Chantal, Nathan, Mike, and Jo for seeing, recognizing, and supporting our crazy ways from the start and enthusing about them.

To the extraordinary people who have influenced, inspired, and guided not only our raw food journey but our lives – Peter, Kerry and Joshua, James and Shelley, Barbara, our raw food mentors Peter Pure, David Wolfe, Gabriel Cousens, and many others.

Lastly, to the Earth, for providing us with everything we need to thrive.

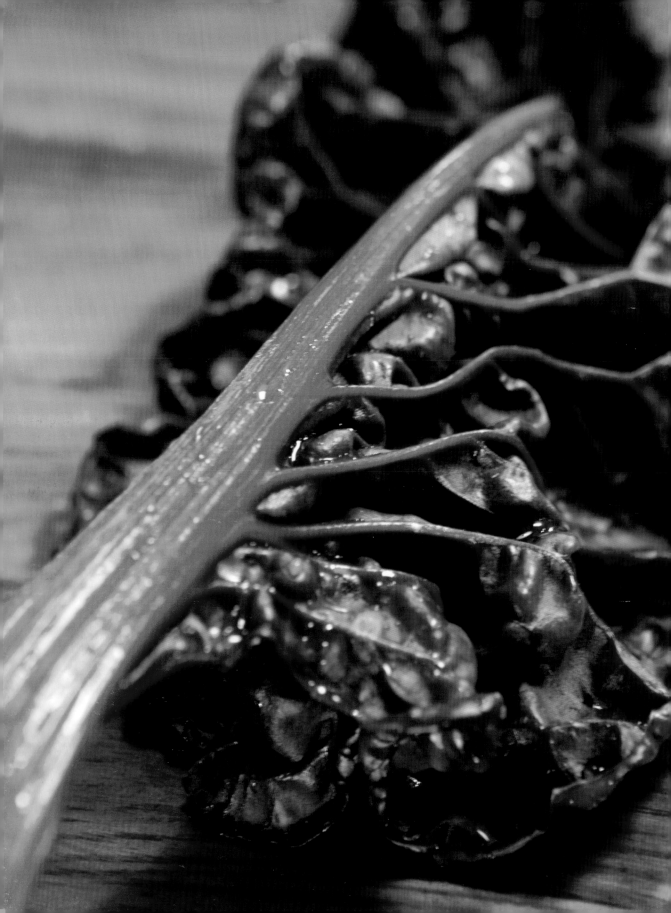

Contents

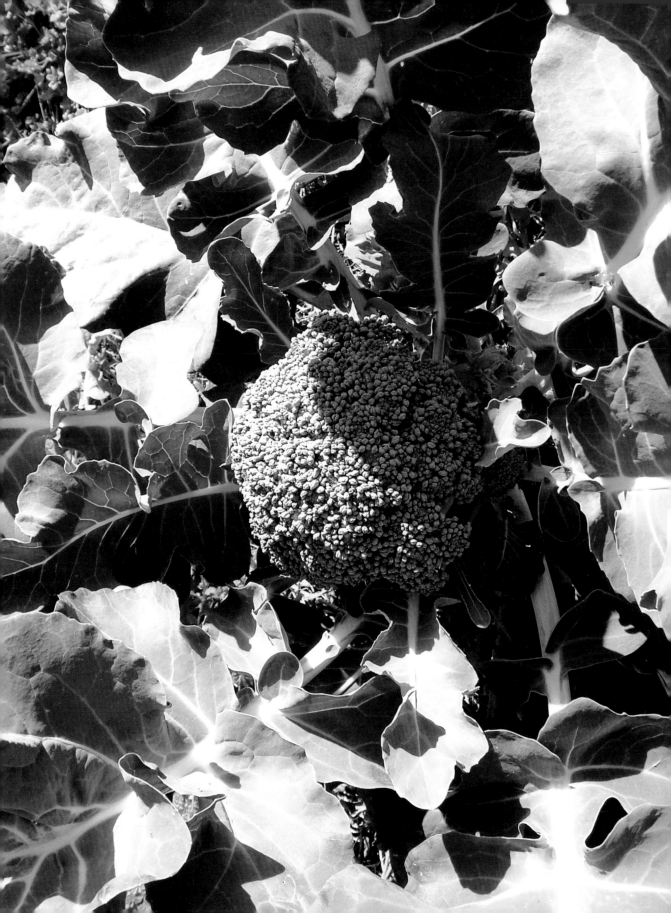

Foreword

Rawlicious is a precious gift to all food lovers who enjoy healthy eating. The book offers a wide spectrum of delicious raw recipes along with a well-written guide to food preparation and is accompanied by gorgeous, breathtaking photographs. The selection of recipes includes soups, salads, dressings, crackers, juices, smoothies, mousses, and cakes, and a wonderful variety of main dishes. The reader can choose from simple recipes that take a few minutes to prepare or more elaborate recipes that will enhance any festive event.

Authors and raw food chefs Peter and Beryn Daniel begin by sharing their insights about the benefits of eating raw, tips on transitioning to a raw food diet, growing sprouts, and more. In the chapter called "Our Raw Food Kitchen," the Daniels provide practical advice about how to stock your kitchen in the most convenient and productive way. Experienced raw food teachers, they then gently escort the reader from one tasty recipe to another.

Rawlicious is richly illustrated with many masterfully done shots of scrumptious dishes and includes photographs of Peter and Beryn growing fruits and vegetables, preparing meals, and enjoying a cup of healthy cheer, which creates the feeling of visiting a young, healthy family and watching them harvest their own produce. Their photographic artistry inspires us to see the beauty of every plant, whether cabbage or sprouts, and even of organic dirt.

Rawlicious is definitely one of the prettiest raw food recipe books in the world. I highly recommend it to anyone interested in raw food.

Victoria Boutenko

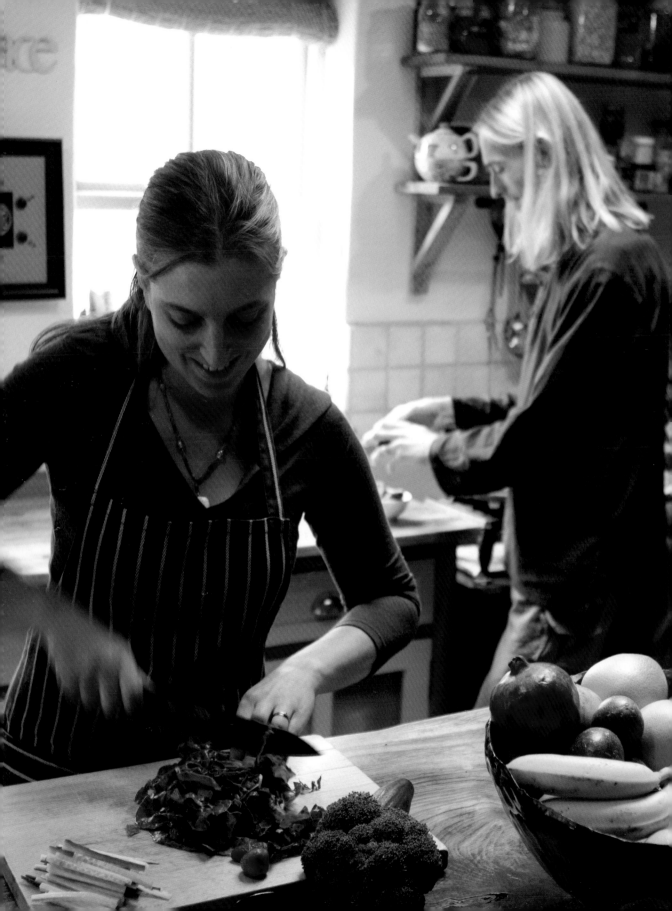

Introduction

This book is the result of an idea whose time has come, an idea that most of us intuitively know and recognize – that to be healthy, happy, naturally nourished, and completely connected to our surroundings is our birthright. After years of eating raw foods and superfoods and running raw food courses, we have met and been inspired by a growing number of people who are becoming aware of the amazing transformative and healing potential of living foods. This book is a natural expression of our experience. We have lived and practiced the concepts and recipes in this book, and continue to do so joyfully.

People are ready to take back responsibility for their health and what they put in their mouths. As raw food chefs, our primary motivation is the long-term health benefits of the food we make and eat. At the same time, we realize that enjoying food is an important and natural part of the experience. If you listen closely you may hear your mother's voice in your head saying, "Don't leave the table until you have finished all your vegetables!" This is probably not the best way to teach someone how to eat healthily. When the food tastes delicious it is easy to eat! "Food" and "health" are two words that should never have been separated. What we have within these pages is a collection of simple, new, and interesting ways to prepare and enjoy raw plant foods.

Peter has written the information sections of this book as a tool to motivate and shift you towards considering a more natural, plant-based diet. Beryn has compiled the recipes that follow to offer practical tools for making delicious food that is truly healthy. This book is an introduction to the topic of raw and living food nutrition. The recommended reading page at the end of the book suggests further reading for those who wish to delve deeper.

Enjoy learning, experimenting, and having fun with your food!

Our Stories

Beryn: My Raw Story

The first recipe I remember learning to make was chocolate sauce. I was six years old. My family has referred to me as a chocoholic for as long as I can remember. Eating Granny's chocolate cake as a midnight feast and again for breakfast was common. My parents owned a bakery and a speciality cake and party shop. I grew up surrounded by cakes, candy, and chocolates. One of my other early childhood memories is of sticking my fingers in chocolate buttercream followed by chocolate sprinkles and licking them clean. My parents were creative, fun, and extravagant in the extreme. For my fourth birthday party I had a train cake mounted on a styrofoam seat that my friends and I could go for rides in. My brother Callan's fourth birthday cake was too big to fit in the front door of our house so we had his party on the front lawn.

What I'm trying to say is that I did not grow up in a family of health freaks. We had fun, we had our cake, and we ate it. And we experienced the side effects. I had suffered with eczema since the age of two but for my family the bigger shock came when my Dad was diagnosed with cancer. I was ten years old. Together, we rollercoasted through hospitals, surgery, chemo, radiation, dietary changes, remission, secondaries, supplements, alternative treatments, and more. My parents were fun and positive, and as a result of having death as a constant and very real advisor, we lived life to the full, traveling all over the world together and having a blast. After being given a 3 percent chance of survival and told to get his affairs in order, my Dad went on to live another eight years. He always used to tell me that the allopathic doctors, nutritionists, and alternative healthcare practitioners needed to learn to work together. Up until the day he died, he was always certain that cancer was not a death sentence. He was right.

When I met Peter we were both nineteen. We got married in 2002 and lived in the UK for a few years, which was where we acquired our first wheatgrass juicer and tried superfoods for the first time. In 2004 we decided to shift direction. We trained together as chefs and began to swing away from any semblance of healthy living. My swing back towards health came fairly swiftly when I next rubbed shoulders with cancer. A friend in London had been diagnosed with breast cancer at the age of forty, three months into her first pregnancy. We moved into their household when her healthy baby boy was just sixteen months old. I took on the role of feeding the family and started to make a more concerted effort to buy organic produce and prepare healthy meals.

During this time, Peter and I did a thirty-day detox challenge. The detox involved excluding all processed foods from our diet – trans fats, wheat, dairy, sugar, alcohol, all animal foods, coffee, and so on. I found myself wandering up and down the supermarket aisles reading labels and putting all my staple canned and bottled ingredients back on the shelves. I ended up in the fruit and vegetable section every time. After the thirty days were over, I felt lighter, clearer, and healthier, but it was at the Vitality Show in London just a few days later that my raw food journey really began. We came across a stall selling raw cakes. The cakes contained only raw ingredients and natural sweeteners; absolutely no wheat, dairy, or flour. Nothing! We bought two slices of cake. I sent Peter back to the stall for two more slices and he signed us up for our first raw chef's training course.

We shifted from a cooked vegan diet to a raw vegan diet over six months. At first, I had an outbreak of eczema which cleared up after about two weeks, never to return. My energy levels skyrocketed. I gained renewed enthusiasm for life and the journey ahead. In the beginning, I would still go back to check whether Granny's chocolate cake really was the best in the world. But eventually, after many months of eating a clean diet, this sugary chocolate cake, the pillar of my childhood days, crumbled. I realized that white refined sugar, wheat, and trans fats really weren't designed for the human organism. I got on with embracing more and more raw food. When we returned home to South Africa, a friend asked us to run a course on healthy eating for her flatmate and friends. This was the beginning of what is now our two-day Raw Food Course.

My journey with raw food continues to unfold. It is an evolving and expanding adventure. I have found that the cleaner my body, the clearer my mind and the more far-reaching my sight. Each day I marvel as horizon after horizon reveals new perceptions and new perspectives, more to learn and more to see. My heart radiates joy as I embrace my passion for living a life in harmony with and connected to the Earth.

Peter: My Raw Story

My interest in food started when I was very young. I remember mixing up all kinds of breakfast cereals to create my own super-muesli when I was just ten years old. Whether it was actually a healthy super-muesli is questionable as, like all my friends, I ate what everyone else around me did without question. The more sugar, chocolate, and potato chips I could get in, the better. I was a fairly sickly youngster, catching colds often and experiencing regular, intense headaches from sinusitis. The gallons of chocolate milk I drank daily were never even considered as the cause. I remember having a box of powdered sugar next to my bed that I would snack on before going to sleep at night! Looking back, I realize I was probably prediabetic. I constantly needed to eat to avoid irritability from low blood sugar and I couldn't hold a glass in one hand without shaking.

Although I did not grow up in a house of health fanatics, my mom believed in home cooking, not takeout food. I learned early to take responsibility for making my own food and this came in very handy when I proposed to Beryn. She said yes on condition that she did not have to cook all the food!

We moved to England, where we attended many health shows as part of our work. This is where I was first introduced to superfoods and juicing. We bought a juicer and juicing soon became part of our routine. In 2004, we decided to train as chefs, working for a while at a French ski resort, where we cooked up five-star gourmet meals that impressed all our guests. During that time I probably ate both better and worse than ever before. The flavors were intoxicating but with all the meat, sugary desserts, and pastries I was eating, the fallout was terrible. I got the flu more times in one year than ever before.

I got my first real wake-up call about nutrition at a powerful motivational event I attended in London. Here I heard things about food that I could not believe. I began researching and found myself being drawn down a rabbit hole. Soon I was training as a raw food chef and diving headlong into nutritional study. I could not believe how little I actually knew about food. No one around me seemed to know anything about the health effects of food, either. The idea that people in this affluent society were dying horrible deaths from degenerative disease caused primarily by poor nutrition was unbelievable to me.

I began testing the concepts by first going off all processed and toxic foods, including animal products. For the first week I was in bed with the worst flu and fever. The initial results of healthy eating did not inspire me much. I stuck with it, however, and made the transition to raw foods over the course of about six months. We moved back to South Africa to focus completely on nutritional study and raw food. The incredible surge of energy and clarity I experienced going raw was channeled into setting up multiple new businesses. I could get away with just four hours of sleep a night and not feel tired. My sinus problems cleared up completely and I felt more vitality and joy than ever before. Friends began to ask questions and soon we were running workshops to teach and pass on our experiences.

My transition to raw was not the result of ill health but of recognizing a way of being that presented incredible opportunities for increased awareness and consciousness. My passion is to refine my experience and explore perception to the highest possible potential, always challenging, questioning, and expanding. The phenomenal changes I've witnessed in myself and in those around me are a constant source of joy and motivation for what I do. I feel honored and blessed to travel my path with heart and to be of service. My greatest wish for you in reading this book is that you are inspired to be more – more joyful, light-hearted, connected, and integrated.

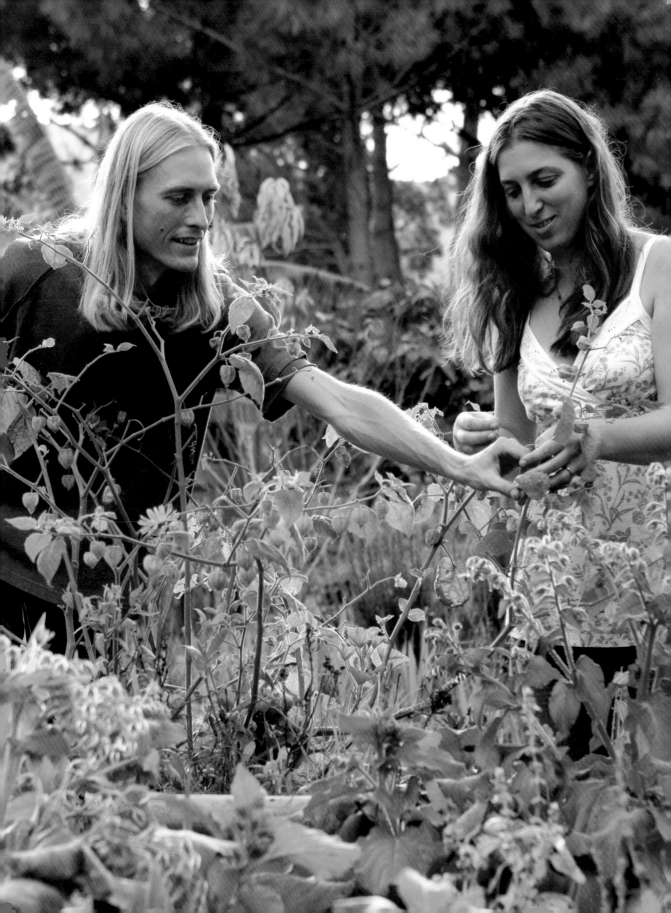

Food and Health

You are what you eat. You may have heard this before; it is one of the most frequently heard statements about food and health. But what does it mean? If you eat nuts, are you nuts? The simplicity of this statement makes it easy to disregard. Our minds are geared towards complexity, yet the most powerful truths are the simplest. What you eat literally becomes you. The nutrients in the food are absorbed and become your cells, blood, tissues, and organs.

Now, if I was building a house to last, I would want to use the best materials available. When it comes to food choices, however, most people treat the building and maintenance of their bodies as though they want to retire in a rundown, dirty, smelly shack. The link between our health and what we eat is irrefutable. The research has been around for decades. I am still amazed at how many people try to argue against the ample evidence in multiple scientific publications. More importantly, we just have to look around us to see the evidence. Are people healthier now than, say, fifty years ago? Do you *not* know someone close to you that has an incurable disease? The statistics are shocking! Our society is crumbling at its core through the cells of the very people it is made up of.

Deadly diseases are steadily on the increase and for all our technological intelligence, there still seem to be no cures. But cures *have* been found. In fact, they have been around for a long time and are used every day to treat and heal diseases that are commonly considered incurable. And the primary healing tool? Nutritional medicine!

When we eat what nature intended – natural whole foods in their original pristine state, un-tampered-with by industry – our bodies heal themselves. Our bodies are designed to regenerate, but without the proper building blocks and nutrients, they cannot. They begin to break down. People worldwide are sick and tired of being sick and tired. Covering up symptoms is not healing. We need to reach for a deeper level of healing. When we truly nourish the body, the body stays healthy.

This is all sounding a bit simple and obvious. So why are more people not using nutritional medicine? Because they have been led to give up their power, specifically their power to choose. I have free choice, don't I? I am not so sure. Consider this: from an early age we are fed processed, sugary junk foods. We are taught that this is food. We grow up watching TV and our young minds, open and highly susceptible to suggestion, have their beliefs about food formed by advertising. Many foods are manufactured to enslave the taste buds. On top of all this, we link childhood emotions to food. Remember ice cream on the beach and getting candy if you were good?

Most minds are truly enslaved. The biggest reason people fail to maintain a healthy lifestyle is not that they don't want to but that they can't undo decades of emotional and mental junk-food programming. The programs *can* be rewritten. Change *is* possible. Growing old with the fear of disease is *not* normal. Health is our natural state of being. It is time to take back our power by accepting that we are responsible for the health of our bodies. It is too late to change once the house has fallen down. What if the first symptom is death?

There are no second chances. There is only today. The choices we make today will affect the health we experience tomorrow. To succeed, one needs to be motivated. Reprogramming takes energy and commitment. Think about what will motivate you to change your diet: Having your children watch you lose your body and mind in old age? Feeling tired all the time? Losing bodily functions? Having to endure painful medical procedures? It *is* possible to choose a different ending to your story.

There is a paradigm shift occurring. Let's now stop looking at the doom and gloom, remove disease from our bodies and minds, and focus instead on what we want. Let's focus on fun, energetic, exciting, and uplifting things. Health food does not have to be boring and bland. Enjoying our food is essential. I enjoy my salads more now than I used to enjoy my junk food meals back when. You can be healthy *and* enjoy your food. The recipes in this book will help you to reprogram and inspire your taste buds and body to return to nature's bounty. Once you are out of the paradigm of disease, avoiding damaging food becomes the obvious way to live. Consciousness expands and true choices are made.

It is true that nothing tastes as good as good health feels, and once you experience the abundant energy, vitality, clarity, strength, and vigor that natural plant-based foods provide, you truly realize how conned most people are. The desire for the junk simply falls away. You begin to eat for life. Remember, disease is not a death sentence, it is simply a wake-up call. The more symptoms you ignore, the louder the body has to shout. Search for answers and look at how your food choices are affecting your body. A healthy lifestyle is simply about removing the poisons and replacing them with the highest-quality nutrition nature has to offer. Give yourself the highest expression and experience of life that you can. The fact that you control what you eat means you have ultimate control over your health.

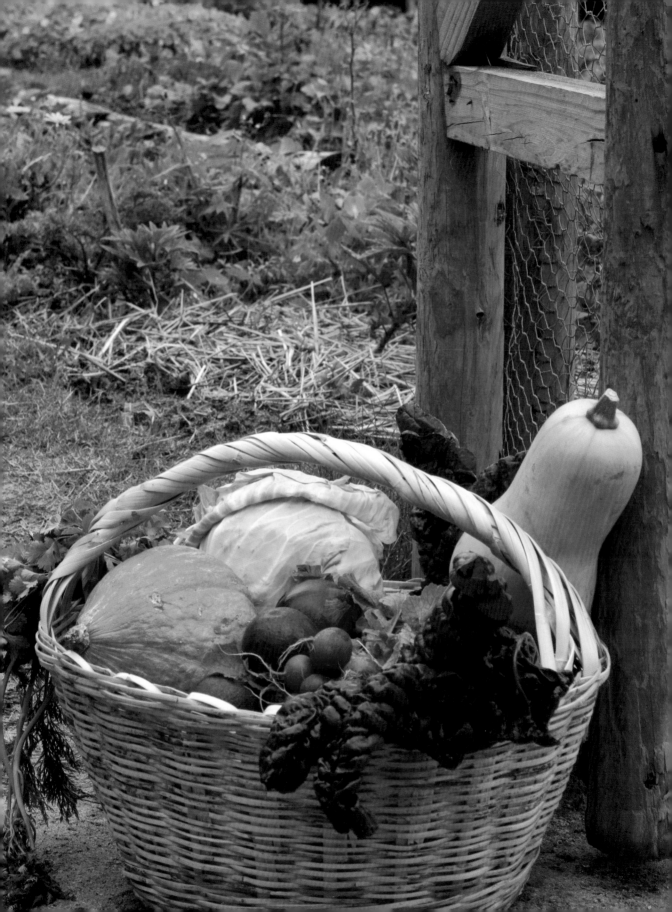

Macro- and Micronutrients

What is food? This may seem like a rhetorical and silly question, but when I see what people put in their mouths I can't help thinking: maybe they don't know what food really is! In our workshops, I've actually found this to be true! People do not know what to eat and why they should eat it. And if that sounds impossible to you, consider these questions:

Is fat bad for cardiovascular health? Is animal protein the best form of protein? Is sugar bad for us? Simple questions that seem to have many conflicting and contradictory answers. But why is feeding ourselves so complicated? Our closest genetic relatives, the chimps, know instinctively and intuitively what to eat for their health and well-being. Are we less intelligent? Let's simplify things.

There are three main food groups, known as macronutrients:
- fats
- carbohydrates
- protein

Within these groups we also have micronutrients:
- vitamins
- minerals
- enzymes
- phytonutrients

The Macronutrients

Fats are an essential part of any healthy and balanced diet. Good fats are raw, plant-based fats. Cooked and processed plant and animal fats promote disease. Whether a fat is saturated or not does not necessarily determine whether it is healthy or unhealthy. Plant-based saturated fat is very different from animal-based saturated fat. Saturated fat is blamed as the cause of cholesterol problems; however, plant fats do *not* contain cholesterol. Animal fats do, and when we eat the cholesterol of an animal we increase our bad cholesterol. In the case of polyunsaturated fats like omega-3 oils, raw marine oils can benefit health if they are free of toxins like mercury, but many seeds such as flax and hemp also contain omega-3 oils. Remember: fat is not bad, it's the *type* that's important. Sources of good fats include olives, olive oil, coconut oil, avocados, nuts, and seeds.

Carbohydrates can also be called sugars. All complex or simple carbohydrates break down to sugar or glucose in the body. Unprocessed natural plant sugars, in their whole-food form, promote health. Processed, refined sugars promote disease. Refined carbs and sugars are one of the most damaging and addictive foods. Refined sugars feed candida, cause metabolic imbalance, and deplete our minerals. The high-sugar, low-mineral Western diet promotes disease. Low-sugar, high-mineral diets are healing. Healthy carbohydrates include fruits, honey, starchy root vegetables, and other vegetables.

Protein is used by the body primarily for repair and maintenance. If you are an uninjured, fully grown adult, you require little protein. We have been led to believe that we need far more protein than we actually do. Animal protein is not superior to plant protein. Amino acids are the building blocks of protein and many plant foods contain complete protein (all essential amino acids). The biggest land animals get *their* complete protein from grass and green leaves! Juicing chlorophyll-rich foods like wheatgrass gives us a potent protein shot. Superfoods like spirulina and hemp seed powder also contain all essential amino acids. At 65 percent protein by weight, spirulina is the highest-protein food on the planet. Other good protein sources include nuts, seeds, olives, green leaves, and certain grains like millet and quinoa. When choosing a vegetarian or vegan diet, it is vital to learn about complete, concentrated plant proteins.

The Micronutrients

The standard Western diet contains far too many macronutrients and not nearly enough micronutrients. Large-scale commercial farming depletes the soil of minerals and life, and the processing and refining of foods reduces their micronutrient content even further. Hunger is the body's search for minerals. Eating loads of macronutrient-rich foods that are deficient in micronutrients does not satiate hunger. Eating lighter, micronutrient-dense foods quickly satisfies the appetite. 95 percent of our body's activities are dependent on minerals, not vitamins. Each cell contains over four thousand enzymes. Those enzymes are only ever fully activated when the major minerals and trace minerals are present in significant quantities. When you feel hungry, it is your body saying, "give me minerals so that I can activate enzymes and make this body function as it should." It is not your body saying, "please stuff in whatever junk you can find so I can spend the rest of the day struggling to digest and eliminate it."

It is virtually impossible to overeat mineral-rich foods. If you're eating mineral-deficient foods you will still feel hungry and tend to overeat. This is not because your body is looking for more of the same mineral-poor foods, but because it hasn't found the minerals it was looking for in the first place!

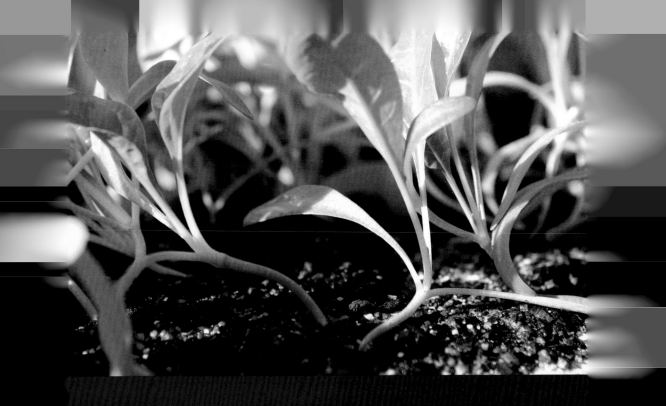

Foods fall into four food quality classes, according to how many minerals they have:

1. Commercially Grown
These are plants that have been hybridized, genetically modified, sprayed with insecticides and pesticides, irradiated, and grown in low quality, demineralized soil.

2. Organic
Organic foods are free from nasty chemicals and sprays and represent foods of a much higher mineral and nutritive value.

3. Homegrown
With homegrown foods you can skyrocket the mineral content of your food by planting in organic soil and adding kitchen leftovers or volcanic rock dust to the soil. Volcanic rock dust is available from any good garden nursery. Plants grown at home with plenty of TLC will grow specifically for you, absorbing the nutrients that you need from the soil to thrive.

4. Wild Plants
On average, wild foods contain fifty times more minerals than commercially grown plants. It's no wonder that in the "old days" cancer, heart disease, and diabetes were virtually unheard of. Our ancestors were living off *wild*, mineral-rich foods.

Physiologically speaking, all disease can be traced back to a mineral deficiency of some kind. When it comes to choosing foods, think about mineral density, and not calories

What Is Raw Food?

Only humans and domesticated animals eat cooked and processed foods. The cooking and processing of food has become so common that most of us do not even consider questioning it. Raw food is plant-based, uncooked food – the way nature provides it to us.

Cooking means heating anything beyond about 116.6°F. Why 116.6°F? At this temperature enzymes in food begin to be destroyed. It is easy to test whether you have breached this temperature threshold – if your finger can't stand the heat, your food can't either. Raw food is not necessarily cold food. Hot teas and soups are great for colder days; just remember to do the finger test for temperature.

What are plant-based foods?
- fruits
- vegetables
- nuts
- seeds
- herbs
- flowers
- leaves
- seaweeds
- superfoods
- sprouts

When you look at what is done to food before it is eaten, you can only conclude that people believe nature has made a mistake. We get fresh, natural food and alter it. Mother Nature does not need to be taught how to feed us. We need to realize that the Earth provides us with everything we need for our time here, and by tampering with what she provides, we compromise the quality of our food and our health.

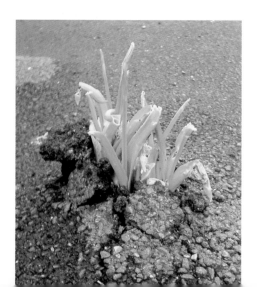

The raw food diet is not actually a diet; it is a lifestyle choice. Most diets leave people feeling deprived and starved. With raw foods, we have the chance to be truly nourished at a deep, cellular level.

Why Eat Raw Foods?

Uncooked foods provide us with more nutrients. The cooking process has been shown to destroy nutrients. The higher the temperature, the more nutrients are destroyed. Low-temperature dehydration is the best method for warming or drying your food. Other forms of cooking such as steaming, boiling, baking, and frying are destructive to the sensitive molecular structure of our food. Most food is cooked at well over 320°F. At such high temperatures up to 80 percent of the nutritional value of food is lost.

Here is a summary of some of the research findings regarding cooking and its effect on food.

- Heat-sensitive vitamins like vitamin C and the B vitamins, including B12, are destroyed.
- Good fats become bad fats and eventually turn into trans fats, the highly toxic type of fat formed in baking and frying.
- 50 percent of the bioavailability of protein is lost when protein-rich foods are cooked.
- A known human carcinogen called acrylamide is formed in the high-temperature cooking of carbohydrates and protein.
- When more than 50 percent of your meal (by weight) is cooked, your body experiences an increased white blood cell count. This means that your immune system has been activated to fight a potential threat: the unrecognizable food you just ate!
- Cooking destroys the electrical charge of the cells of our food. Our cells in turn lose their charge and can't function properly.
- Red blood cells clump together and can't efficiently carry oxygen or detoxify the body.

Because of the destruction of all enzymes, cooked food requires far more energy to digest. Animal foods, especially meat, are considered the most energetically draining to try and digest.

Cooking also increases the acid-forming nature of food. Our internal acid-alkaline balance is one of our primary health balances. If our bodies become too acidic, disease follows. If our bodies are alkaline, disease cannot take hold. We are not only acidified by food; stress, environmental toxins, medication, dehydration, and negative emotional states all have an acidic effect.

Alkaline-forming foods include green leaves, sprouts, sea vegetables, non-sweet fruits, vegetables grown above the ground, and certain grains like millet and buckwheat.

Acid-forming foods include root veggies, nuts, seeds, and sweet fruits. Highly acid-forming foods are usually animal-based foods and highly processed plant foods. Some of the worst acidic offenders are: meat products, refined sugars, trans fats (including hydrogenated fats), refined carbs including sugar, wheat and maize flour, cow's milk, highly processed soy foods like burgers and sausages, fizzy drinks, artificial sweeteners, and coffee. Most food eaten in the Western diet is acid-forming. Correcting this imbalance is one of the most important steps you can take to ensure long-lasting health. It is beyond the scope of this book to go into detail about pH balance and health and why certain foods are so toxic. I urge you to question and do some research to educate yourself about these poisonous "foods."

Many people are allergic to refined wheat, gluten, sugar, and dairy in some way, but for those who have been diagnosed with a related condition or intolerance, dietary options often feel limited and restrictive. Adopting a raw food approach is an obvious choice because of the lack of offending allergens, but what's more, eating this way is fun.

Green leaves have the greatest ability to heal and correct pH imbalance. Juicing greens daily is a powerful health tool. The juicing section offers further information and recipes to get you going.

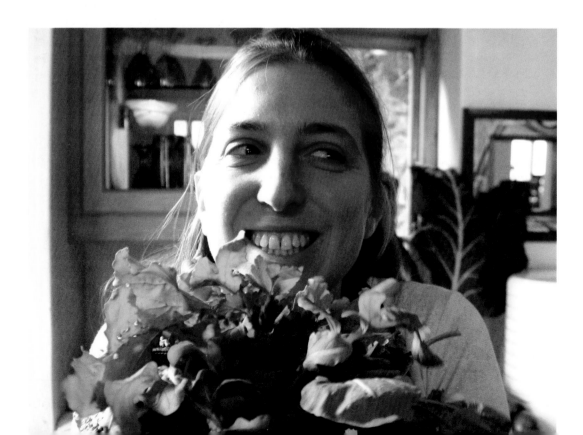

The Benefits of Eating Raw

There is a big difference between information and knowledge. What you are reading now is simply information. If you test out these concepts and practice the principles, you will have personal experience, which is knowledge. The benefits of eating a plant-based raw diet are many, but until you experience them for yourself they are just stories. This is what I love about raw nutrition – you simply have to eat to experience the benefits! Some people experience major positive change within days.

From the previous chapters you already have some idea of the positive results of going raw, but I will briefly mention some of the benefits Beryn and I have experienced personally, and feedback we have received from people who have embraced a raw lifestyle. I want to emphasize that although this list of benefits may seem miraculous, they are simply by-products of a well-nourished body. Every person is also at a unique level of wellness and will experience different results over a period of time. It can take a number of years to truly correct the extreme nutritional deficiencies acquired over decades.

One of the most common benefits of going raw is a feeling of lightness and clarity. It's as if a cloud lifts off the mind. Emotions become more stable; it becomes easy to smile for no apparent reason. A sense of anxiousness and uncertainty vanishes and is replaced by a calm, centered confidence and feeling of connectedness. On a physical level, many chronic conditions show remarkable improvement and true healing occurs. The quality of skin, nails, and hair improves. Recovery time from exercise greatly improves and stamina and strength increase. The body naturally and easily releases excess weight. Many people experience dramatic results with weight loss. Less sleep is required, because the body is no longer detoxifying all night long. You produce far less garbage at home as your peels become compost. Colds and flu become a thing of the past. Your body is able to adjust to changing seasonal temperatures more easily. You eat less food as hunger is truly satiated – the list goes on and on.

Our potential for health and wellness is truly awesome. Act, experience, and know!

Health Is Not All About Food

Food is an important part of health but we must be clear that it is only a part. A holistic approach to health is required, taking other factors such as water, air, exercise, emotions, and mental state into consideration.

Our bodies are made up mostly of water and constantly need to maintain hydration. Drinking enough clean water is essential; if you don't filter your faucet water, *you* are the filter! We exclusively drink spring water that we collect from the source and store in glass. The Earth is the ultimate water filter and true springs offer the purest and best water to drink. How much water you should drink in a day depends on many factors, such as exercise, your toxicity levels, and the amount of water-rich foods eaten. If you can start your day with a pint of water, you are well on your way to hydration. Get a glass bottle and keep water with you throughout the day.

Breathing can easily be taken for granted. Due to stressful lifestyles people tend to breathe in a shallow way, and don't use the abdomen to inhale fully and deeply. The air quality in most cities is another concern. Go for walks in nature often and practice breathing exercises to get more oxygen into your system.

Regular exercise creates a strong, fit body, allows detoxification through sweating, and builds healthy bones. Sitting at a desk all day just won't make you energetic and vibrant. Get moving!

Our mind and emotions can be our greatest healing tool or our downfall. It is incredible how powerful the mind is and how much can be achieved with the right thinking. Focus on the positive, don't dwell on the negative. Negative thoughts and emotions are acidic to the body.

If you drink clean water, eat loads of raw, mineral-rich food, breathe deeply, get out and breathe in the fresh air often, and move your body, you will have a finely tuned system that will give you an energetic, quality ride! Top it all off with enjoying what you do and having positive, empowering thoughts, and you have the recipe not only for health and well-being but for joy, love, and abundance on all levels.

Transitioning to Raw Foods

The beginning is a very delicate time. Your body is adjusting to new foods, detoxifying old garbage, and repairing years of neglect. For most people, it is more appropriate to start slowly, gradually increasing the amount of raw food and decreasing the amount of cooked food you eat than to go 100 percent raw overnight. It takes a little bit of time to unravel preconceptions about food, not to mention all the emotional attachments to various foods. We call it the gradient principle. If you try and jump to the top of a flight of stairs in one leap you will probably hurt yourself and fall back down. Take it one step at a time, and suddenly you are at the top. Transition at a pace you can maintain and sustain. Don't be too relaxed about it either, though. Get out of your comfort zone but not into your shock zone.

Two other powerfully simple principles for transitioning are:
- the Just Add In principle
- the Just Take Out principle

With the Just Add In principle, the idea is to simply add in new raw foods, without necessarily even changing your normal diet. So, if you are a bacon-and-eggs-for-breakfast kind of person, just add in a pint of green-vegetable juice before you have breakfast. If you snack on junk food during the day, first have a handful of goji-and-cacao trail mix. This is a natural way of pushing out the bad without forcing the change. The nutrient-dense raw food will make you so full you won't want to eat the other stuff.

The Just Take Out principle acknowledges that if you tell a child not to do something, they *will* do it. If you tell an adult not to do or eat something, they will do or eat it when no one is looking! So instead of forcing yourself to give up junk food, take on the thirty-day "just take out" challenge: For thirty days, commit to completely removing certain foods from your diet. Wheat, dairy, trans fats, and sugar are good places to start. It's only for thirty days! This principle works by allowing the body's internal feedback system to reawaken. Our bodies are amazing machines. They will cope with incredible stress and poisoning but when we give them a break and let them recover, adding the "poison food" back in after thirty days usually causes an instant, often projectile detox response! The body has gotten used to the poison, but cutting it out for thirty days and then adding it back in gives you a chance to feel its full effect. Look out for phlegm, tiredness, irritability, and headaches. A word of warning with this one: if you eat the "poison" three times within a day or two after the thirty days, you will be hooked again and your body will revert to its old state of coping with the situation.

During or after the thirty days, you might find you give in and eat the thing you are trying to cut out. When this happens it is very important to use the experience to gain new knowledge. See it as an experiment. Notice any mental, emotional, or physical changes you may have. Do not say things like "I cheated" or "it was an accident." These words are rooted in guilt, which is a powerful acidic emotion that will probably cause more harm than the food you just ate.

Lifeboat Supplements for Cooked Foodists

There are a few supplements that are very beneficial for transitioning:

Digestive enzymes
Eating cooked food depletes the body's store of enzymes until you eventually can't digest food properly anymore. Adding in supplemental plant-based enzymes will support your digestive system, enabling it to properly absorb your food. Initially, it's best to take them with every meal you eat and gradually move on to only having them when you eat cooked food. The cooked food has no enzymes left to help you digest it. The effect of using enzymes can be noticed immediately.

Probiotics
Probiotics are good bacteria, also known as our allied army of defense. They should line your entire digestive system and number in the trillions. However, because of factors such as antibiotics, drinking chlorinated water, eating meat, radiation exposure, stress, and drinking alcohol, they get destroyed. When our good guys are dead and gone, the bad guys grow and take over. Candida, yeast, molds, and fungus thrive in this environment and a breeding ground for worms and bacteria is created, which ultimately compromises the digestive and immune systems. Take a good, quality probiotic supplement regularly. The more you are exposed to the things that destroy probiotics, the more often you will need to take them. Cultured foods such as sauerkraut and kimchi, as well as fermented nut cheeses, are also a great source of good bacteria.

Greens
Greens are probably the most important food group. They are rich in chlorophyll, alkalizing minerals, and sun energy. Concentrated superfood green powders are one of the easiest ways to get more greens into your diet. The best source is grasses, with barleygrass and wheatgrass being the most common. Take green powder supplements daily to boost your alkaline minerals.

Detoxing

When you begin to transition into eating raw you will most likely experience a healing crisis, or detoxification episodes. When we stop poisoning our system, it has a chance to dump all the toxic buildup from the tissues and lymphatic system. The experience can be uncomfortable, with symptoms ranging from headaches, nausea, diarrhea, dizziness, aches, and pains to rashes, mucus discharge, fatigue, and irritability. It's important to remember that it's not the food that is doing it to you, it's the elimination of the old junk and the release of the related toxic buildup. Drinking plenty of water and green-vegetable juices is helpful, as is getting lots of rest. Detox episodes should not last more than a few hours to a few days at a time. If you feel ill for a week or more, make sure you don't have a food intolerance to something you have added in, and go to your homeopath or holistic doctor for assistance.

Cleansing is a necessary part of life and even if we have the best diet, living in cities toxifies us. Regular juice feasts, where you fast on green-vegetable juice, are a powerful way to detoxify. Further cleansing can include colon hydrotherapy, herbal colon cleanses, and other herbal organ cleanses. The colon is the first place to start, and daily cleansing is a great way to limit toxic buildup. Drinking green-vegetable juice, eating fiber-rich salads, taking supplements like zeolites, enzymes, MSM, and probiotics will make up an effective daily protocol. A yearly parasite flush is also a good idea. Parasites live in impacted fecal matter stuck to the folds of the colon from processed, fiberless foods. They sap your energy and excrete toxins of their own into our systems. A good herbal parasite remedy including black walnut hulls, cloves, and wormwood should be taken for at least ninety days to make sure that all the eggs that hatch are destroyed. Cleansing is not a quick fix. It can take years of eating well and cleansing regularly to clear out most of the toxic load, but every step yields results that are clearly felt.

Planning for Success

If you don't have a plan, you're following someone else's plan! Setting up your day to succeed by planning your meals is an excellent tool for transitioning. If you start off your day by making a green vegetable juice and a smoothie, and put them in flasks to drink throughout the day, you are off to a great start. Have a big salad for lunch, and snack on superfood trail mixes and fruit. If you do this you will find you are suddenly eating over 70 percent raw already! It's really that simple. If you make a weekly meal plan and shop to it accordingly, you won't be duped by advertising and packaging trying to get you to buy on impulse. Look for new places to buy organic produce and products. There is most likely even an option for you to shop online and avoid the supermarkets altogether.

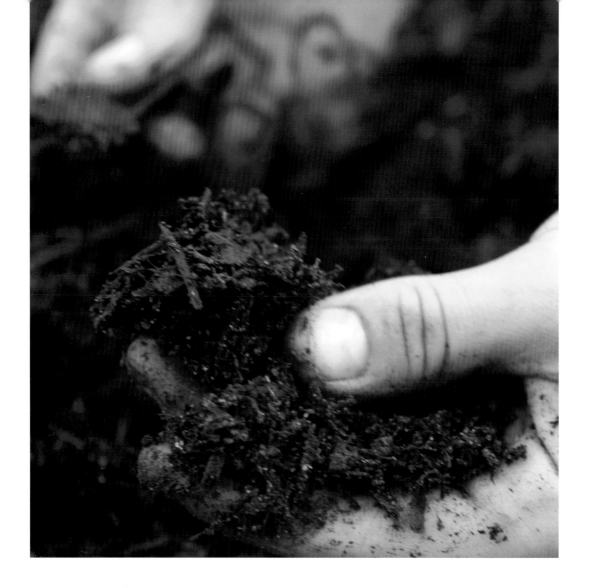

Connecting to the Earth

One of the simplest and most effective practices for good health is taking off your shoes and getting connected to the Earth, barefoot. The planet is constantly releasing electrons that provide potent antioxidant benefits. Being insulated in rubber shoes and concrete or wooden houses prevents us from connecting to this natural force. Another huge benefit of being barefoot daily, even if just for a few minutes, is that you ground (neutralize) any electromagnetic "smog" that's gotten stuck to you throughout the day. The results of this simple practice are truly magical, and you may not want to put your shoes back on again!

Succeeding on a Raw Food Diet

Ratio Is Key

You can be unhealthy on a raw food diet. A healthy diet is as much about balancing the food groups as it is about choosing the highest quality foods available. Balance is about ratio. The ratio is between how many carbs, fats, and greens you are ingesting. It is easy to overdo the fats and sugars. Reducing the amount of sugars initially by going on a low- to no-sugar diet will accelerate healing. Eating fat is comforting and a big dietary shift can be unsettling, so overeating fat is common, too. However, too many fats can make you feel sluggish and tired and put stress on your liver. The biggest mistake people initially make on a raw diet is avoiding greens. Greens can form as much as half of your diet, providing protein, alkalizing minerals, and fiber. If you aren't feeling great, look at how you've been doing with the ratio of carbs to fats to greens.

Getting Support

Changing your diet without the support of friends and family is probably the most challenging aspect of going raw. Your loved ones won't know what you know and will be concerned for your health. If they are open to it, give them as much information as possible. There is no need to be defensive or aggressive about your dietary choices; don't make it an issue and it won't be. People are usually just unsure of what to feed you when you visit, so ease their discomfort by explaining that it's actually much simpler to feed a raw foodist and that you are happy to bring your own snacks, a salad, or even a healthy raw dessert. If you are secure and confident in your choices and you enjoy what you eat there will be no need for people to try and change your mind. Remember that if you judge others for what they eat they will judge you for what you eat. We all want the best health for our friends and family but if you are preachy and antagonistic, you will not get a positive result. Be supportive and understanding, allowing each person to travel their own path whilst being ready to assist and give advice when asked. Regularly getting together with others who are interested in raw foods creates an excellent support structure. Organize weekly or monthly raw food dinners and get everyone to bring a recipe and a dish.

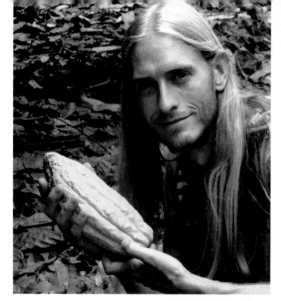
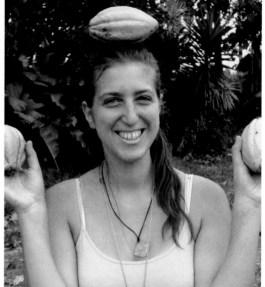

Superfoods

Superfoods are the new technology available to us for achieving the best health ever! It's actually a really old technology, as most ancient cultures from around the world have certain foods that they revere more than others. Superfoods can be seen as whole food supplements, something between a food and a herb. They are foods that are exceptionally rich in nutrient density and offer incredible healing potential. In order to address the huge nutritional deficit we have accumulated over decades, we need a secret weapon – something to give us an extra boost back to health and vitality. That is exactly why superfoods are becoming so popular; people eat them and notice a difference. Popping pills that cost a fortune and yield no noticeable results except for yellow urine day after day is crazy. We are incredibly fortunate to have a large selection of superfoods available for us to try.

These are some of our top superfoods:
- *Goji berries:* the Chinese super-berry for longevity.
- *Raw cacao:* all chocolate comes from the cacao bean, which grows in the jungle in large pods. This truly healthy chocolate provides heaps of antioxidants, minerals, and mood-enhancing nutrients.
- *Maca:* Peruvian power-food for building stamina, vitality and hormones.
- *Hemp seed protein:* an easily digestible complete protein source.
- *Spirulina:* the wonder algae – super high in protein and chlorophyll.
- *Barley and wheatgrass*: nutrient powerhouse for alkalizing.
- *Coconut oil:* healthy saturated fat for energy.

For more information on these and other superfoods, visit our website at www.superfoods.co.za.

Try them out and find the ones that work for you.

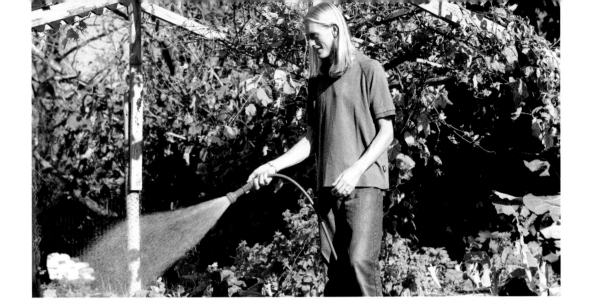

Growing Your Own Food

If there is one thing you can do to transform not only your own health but the health of the planet, it's growing your own food. Nurturing a garden and reaping the harvest of your own labor of love is one of the most rewarding things you can do. Not only do homegrown foods provide you with superior nutrition, you can grow them without chemicals and pesticides, and they taste much better than anything you can buy! There is a great deal of joy, security, and confidence that comes from knowing you can feed yourself by your own hand. This is one of the most fundamentally important life skills, yet few people know how to grow their own food! The fear of starvation is a very real subconscious fear for most people, and rightly so. If you rely on others to feed you, you have no food security.

Growing your own food can be as simple or complex as you like. From large veggie patches to veggie pots to indoor sprouting, there is an option for everyone. There are excellent workshops you can attend to learn how to create your own organic food garden.

Sprouting

One of the quickest ways to get started is to get sprouting. Sprouts are super easy to grow and incredibly nutritious. Buying sprouts from shops can be up to ten times more expensive than growing your own. Sprouts are one of nature's true living superfoods – they are enzyme-rich, high in amino acid (protein) content, bursting with minerals and trace minerals, and are packed with chlorophyll. Sprouts are also healing and therapeutic, cleansing and alkalizing, and filled with antiaging antioxidants. Because they are so high in minerals and enzymes, they facilitate digestion, detoxification, and weight loss. What's more, they taste fantastic. There is a wide selection of different types of seeds that one can sprout, so the variety and flavors available are virtually endless.

The Glass Jar Method

There are many different sprouting kit options, ranging from stackable plastic rings to glass jars, sprouting bags, and automatic sprouters. My favorite is the glass jar method. Sprouting with this simple system involves soaking your chosen seeds overnight and covering the jar with a mesh screen and rubber band. In the morning drain the soak water and rinse the seeds twice daily, placing them on a rack to drain during the day. Harvest them within three to seven days. Some of the easiest sprouts to grow are alfalfa, fenugreek, radish, broccoli, mung beans, onion, cabbage, mustard seeds, chickpeas, quinoa, lentils, pea sprouts, and wheat seeds. For most sprouts, continue to sprout them until they have developed a long tail or their first leaves have begun to go green. In the case of chickpeas, quinoa, pea sprouts, and lentils, they are ready to eat as soon as their tails begin to unfurl or emerge from the seed.

Sprouting Buckwheat

Buckwheat is a very versatile seed that has many uses in raw dishes. Sprouting buckwheat takes a little more attention. Soak the seeds overnight in a glass jar. In the morning rinse thoroughly. Place the seeds in a large bowl or glass jar and cover with a dish towel. Allow to sprout for one to two days. The sprouts are ready as soon as the little tail has emerged from the seed. Buckwheat releases a gelatinous substance that needs to be rinsed away thoroughly in order to avoid mold.

Soil-grown Microgreens

Another way of growing sprouts is directly in soil trays. These kind of sprouts are called microgreens. My favorites are wheatgrass, barleygrass, or sunflower greens.

How to grow soil-based sprouts:
- Buy trays and organic growing soil from a garden nursery.
- Fill the trays with soil.
- Soak wheat, barley, or sunflower seeds overnight.
- Drain them in the morning and allow them to stand in a bowl for 24–48 hours.
- Small tails will sprout.
- Place the seeds on top of the soil, cover with another thin layer of soil, and lightly water them.
- Place them in an area that gets either the morning or afternoon sun (midday summer sun will burn the young shoots) and water daily.
- Harvest the wheatgrass or barleygrass after seven to ten days and juice it.
- Harvest the sunflower sprouts after seven to ten days and either juice them or eat them in salads.

To provide your soil-grown sprouts with a full complement of minerals and trace minerals, take Himalayan rock salt and make a salt-water solution of one part salt to 200 parts water. Water the sprouts from day four to day seven with this salt-water solution. Alternatively, get sea water (from a clean source, preferably a few miles out to sea) and make the solution from one part sea water to 20 parts fresh water and proceed as before. You will have the healthiest looking, best-tasting, super-nutritious sprouts around.

Remember that sprouting is not just about growing your own food – it's about reestablishing a communication with the plant world and also the Earth. It's about reconnecting with your own creative ability and taking the time each day to do something truly supportive for yourself.

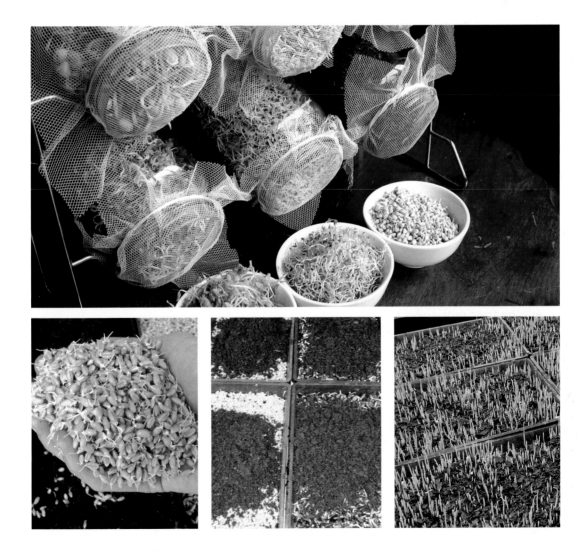

Using this Recipe Book

Rawlicious is about having fun with your food. It is about cultivating an awareness for consciously choosing quality ingredients and preparing them with love.

A summary of what you will need

- a generous handful of fun
- a touch of laughter
- a dash of action
- 2–4 pints (1–2 L) of spring water
- 2 pints (1 L) of green vegetable juice
- fresh air
- lots of healthy, delicious, fresh, raw, and organic produce
- a cupboard full of superfoods
- a sprinkling of awesome company
- a big dollop of joy

Mix together vigorously and tuck in.

All the recipes in this book are a guideline and a springboard to get your own creative juices flowing. Rules are meant to be broken and so are recipes. Taste, adjust, taste again, and experiment with the outlines set out in this book. Remember to have fun and play with your food. Smile, laugh, dance, and sing while you're preparing your meals.

Conversion Table

1 cup	250 ml	8 fl. oz
1/2 cup	125 ml	4 fl. oz
1/3 cup	80 ml	3 fl. oz
1/4 cup	60 ml	2 fl. oz
1/8 cup	30 ml	1 fl. oz

Suns and Fact Files

On many of the recipe pages you will see a sun with writing – this will contain facts about one or more of the ingredients used in the dish on that page and why it is good for you.

Sticky Notes

On other pages you will find sticky notes – preparation notes to remind you of pre-prep factors to take into account when getting ready to make the raw dish on that page.

Ingredients

- Begin reading labels. If you don't understand or cannot pronounce the words on the label, it's normally best to leave it on the shelf where you found it.
- "Fresh ingredients" – i.e., organic or homegrown wherever possible; juices are freshly squeezed and water is ideally from a natural spring.
- Herbs and spices should be nonirradiated and preferably organic.
- Oils are extra virgin, cold pressed, and organic.
- Salt is Himalayan rock salt or unbleached, non-iodized sea salt.
- Soy-based sauces such as tamari or Bragg Liquid Aminos must be organic and non-GM (genetically modified).
- All dried fruits are preservative- and sulfur dioxide-free.
- All cacao is raw and all honey is raw and unheated.
- Maple syrup is pure Canadian maple syrup and not maple-flavored syrup.
- "Hot water" is parboiled water that has not been heated over 158°F.
- All pasteurized foods have been avoided as this means they have been cooked.

Other Actions

Juicing: pressing your own fresh produce through a single- or twin-gear masticating juicer to extract your own freshly squeezed juice.

Blending: using a high-speed or power blender to make up smoothies, pâtés, sauces, soups, and desserts.

Dehydrating: using a dehydrator to dry or warm foods slowly at under 116.6°F.

Spiralizing: using a spiralizer to make vegetable noodles.

Mandolining: using a mandolin to cut julienne strips or thin slices of various vegetables.

Our Raw Food Kitchen

A raw food kitchen has some markedly different features to a standard cooking kitchen. For example, our oven is switched off at the mains and we use it for storing shopping bags; the stovetop is covered with baskets of fresh produce.

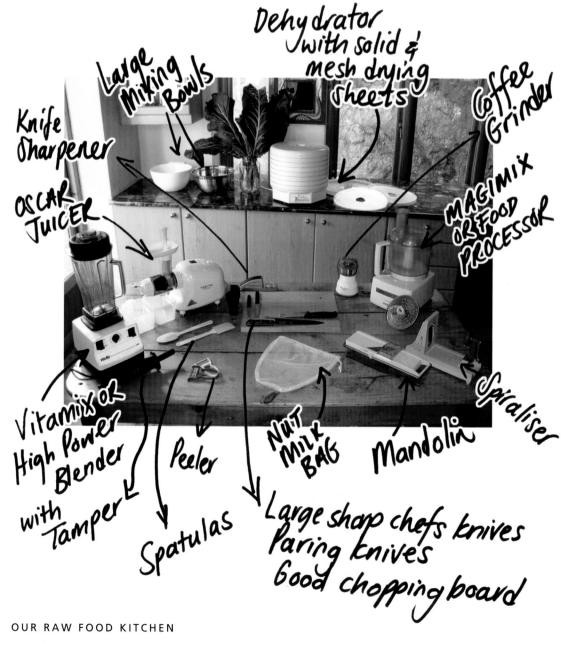

Dehydrator with solid & mesh drying sheets

Large Mixing Bowls

Knife Sharpener

OSCAR JUICER

Coffee Grinder

MAGIMIX OR FOOD PROCESSOR

Vitamix or High Power Blender with Tamper

Peeler

Spatulas

NUT MILK BAG

Mandolin

Spiraliser

Large sharp chefs knives
Paring knives
Good chopping board

Setting up a raw kitchen can at first glance seem expensive. Firstly, I would recommend changing your perspective. Disease is a far riskier and more expensive business than health. What may seem like a hefty investment now is more than likely going to save you heaps in the long term, not to mention ensure that you are around with all your faculties intact to see the long term. Secondly, I would suggest setting up your kitchen in stages. You may find that some of the tools you already have can double up in the meantime for ones you want to start saving for. For example, a hand blender or simple smoothie blender can make most of the smoothies described in this book. The food processor can make most of the sauces. However, the power blender gives you more versatility and the dehydrator takes raw fooding to a whole new level. Eventually, you are going to want to own all the equipment and superfoods that make this lifestyle simple and fun, but do it at a pace that is right for you and your budget.

Kitchen Essentials:
A large, sharp chef's knife
Paring knives
Knife sharpener
Chopping board
Spatulas
Peeler

Kitchen Equipment:
Juicer
Power blender
Dehydrator with extra solid and mesh sheets
Food processor with S-blade and grating attachments

Kitchen Accessories:
Nut milk bag
Mandolin
Spiralizer
Coffee grinder
Large stainless-steel mixing bowls
Measuring cups
Measuring spoons
Colander
Flat pallet knife
Glass storage jars with your favorite nuts, seeds, and superfoods clearly displayed.

For more information on kitchen equipment and where to get the best machines, see the resources section at the back of this book.

Stocking your Kitchen

Step 1: Clear out your cupboards.

Before you get started with the task of stocking your kitchen for raw success, you have to undertake the task of *de*-stocking your kitchen. Yes, we're talking about cupboard clearing. Just do it! Those pastas and box milks that have been sitting in the corners gathering dust need not take up your valuable shelf space.

Step 2: Restock with the good stuff. (Below is a list of kitchen essentials you'll usually find in our kitchen.)

Step 3: Throw out your microwave.

Step 4: Put your toaster at the back of the cupboard.

Step 5: Give your new juicer or blender prime space on the kitchen counter!

Spices & seasoning:	Seeds:	Oils:
Cumin	Flax or linseeds	Organic olive oil
Cilantro	Sunflower seeds	Hemp oil
Cinnamon	Pumpkin seeds	
Curry masala	Sesame seeds	Nuts:
Cayenne pepper	Sprouting seeds:	A variety of raw nuts:
Turmeric	*mung beans, alfalfa,*	*almonds, walnuts, cashews,*
Mixed herbs	*adzuki, lentils, fenugreek,*	*macadamias, pine nuts,*
Dulse flakes	*cabbage, mustard,*	*Brazil nuts, pecans*
Kelp	*Japanese radish, broccoli,*	
Himalayan rock salt	*chickpeas*	

Grains:
Quinoa

Seaweed:
Whole dulse leaf
Wakame
Nori sheets

Outside in the garden or in trays:
Sunflower seed sprouts
Wheatgrass

Other savory essentials:
Garlic bulbs
Ginger
Red onions
Chillies
Lemons
Organic tamari sauce
Tahini
Apple cider vinegar
Organic coconut milk
Sundried tomatoes
Black olives

Other sweet selections:
Agave nectar
A variety of raw honeys
Organic coconut flakes
Raisins
Dates
Dried figs
Dried mango
Raw muesli

Superfoods:
Bee pollen
Raw cacao powder
Raw cacao beans
Raw cacao nibs
Raw cacao butter
Goji berries
Maca powder
Hemp protein powder
Spirulina powder
Green powder mix
Yacon root powder
Lacuma powder
Coconut oil

Water:
For drinking, I collect water from the local spring and fill a 6 gallon (25 L) glass container.
I filter all the water that comes into my house with a Big Blue water filtration system, so that even the bath and shower water is clean.

Fresh produce:
I usually shop twice a week for fresh produce – once online from the Ethical Co-op and once from my local organic produce store or health shop

My fresh shopping usually includes:
A selection of salad greens
Arugula
Mustard greens
Cucumbers for juicing
Celery for juicing
Apples or grapefruit
Spinach or swiss chard
Red or green cabbage
Carrots
Zucchini
Eggplant
Broccoli or cauliflower
Tomatoes
Avocados
Beetroots
Red peppers
Basil
Cilantro
Parsley
Mangos
Papaya
Passion Fruit
Bananas
Butternut squash
Yams
Fresh figs
Pomegranates
Blueberries
Raspberries
Other fresh seasonal fruit

Supplements:
MSM
Digestive enzymes
Methylcobalamin-B12
Probiotic powder
Anti-parasitic formula

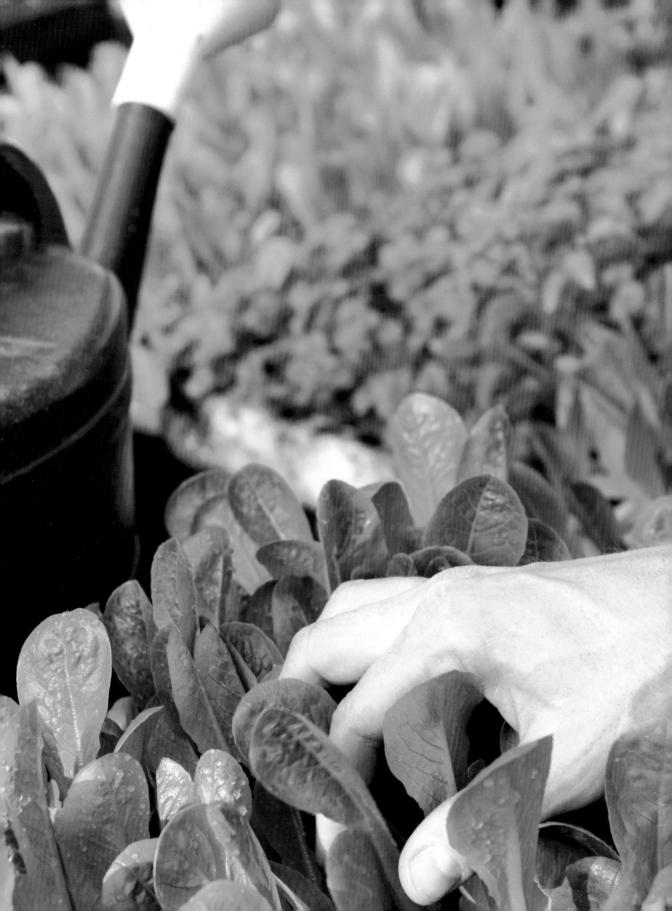

Juices
Liquid Elixirs

Ten Reasons to Juice

Our juice recipes are based around green vegetable juicing. There are many reasons for this. Here are our top ten.

1. Cleansing and Alkalizing
Green leafy vegetables and grasses are the most cleansing and alkalizing to the body. By juicing them you are giving your body what it needs to balance your pH level and keep yourself in optimal health.

2. Enzymes
Freshly extracted juices are the best source of live enzymes.

3. Nutrients, vitamins, and minerals
Juiced vegetables provide your body with high amounts of absorbable chlorophyll, amino acids, minerals, vitamins, and phytonutrients.

4. Easier to digest and absorb
Juicing takes the strain off the digestive system. By extracting the juice from the fiber, it predigests the fruits and vegetables for you, making the nutrients more readily available for easy absorption. Fiber in the diet is important, though, so drink your vegetables and eat your fruit.

5. Easier to consume
Years of eating nutritionally deficient food means that a lot of alkalizing green foods are needed to rebalance our bodies. We couldn't eat enough greens to address this imbalance. Juicing provides a simple and effective way to get maximum goodness into the body without having to graze on grass all day long.

6. True hydration
The planet is over 70 percent water and so are our bodies. Our blood consists of around 94 percent water. Foods in their natural and raw state have a high water content. By drinking these water-rich fruit and vegetable juices we can ensure and enjoy proper hydration.

7. Antioxidants
Green juice provides the body with huge amounts of antioxidants. Antioxidants fortify our immune systems and stop our bodies rusting from the inside out.

8. Delivers oxygen to your cells

When our bodies are acidic the red blood cells clump together and oxygen cannot get to all the cells. Juicing alkalizes the blood so that the red blood cells can flow freely once again and deliver oxygen to each and every cell in your body. When your body is charged with oxygen your mind is clear and sharp and you feel energized.

9. Disease prevention

It is no coincidence that strong therapeutic green vegetable, sprout, and grass juices form the cornerstone of every successful disease prevention center and clinic around the world.

10. Calming

The magnesium and chlorophyll in green juices soothes and calms the nervous system and minimizes stress in the body.

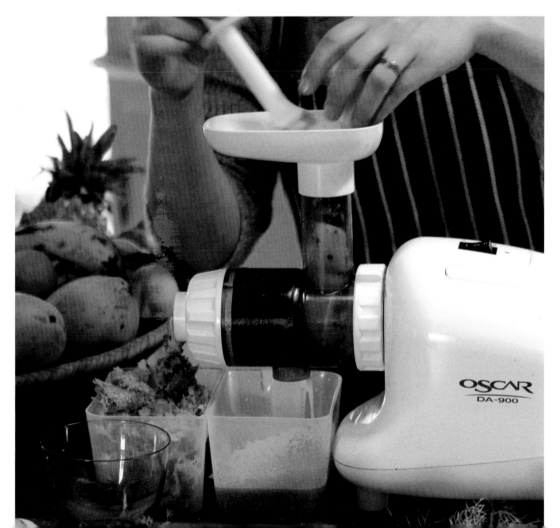

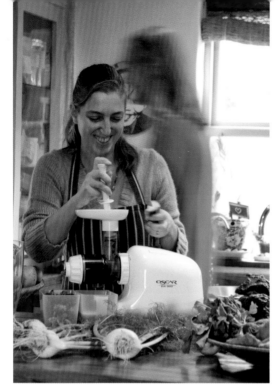
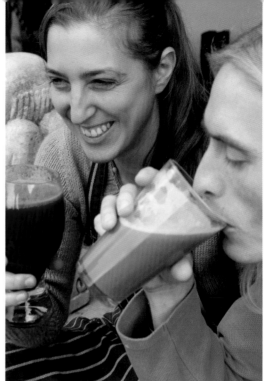

The Basics of Juicing

I am going to expand on the basics for a moment because I really want you to get how important it is to start juicing your vegetables. If all you do after you put down this book is start green vegetable juicing, I can assure you your body is going to thank you with longer-lasting health.

How often should I juice?
Every day.

How much should I drink in a day?
1 quart of green vegetable juice. It is a good idea to dilute your juice. Juice yourself 1 pint and then dilute with 1 pint water to make up your 1 quart for the day.

When should I juice?
In the morning is best, so that you can start your day off with a fresh glass and sip on the rest throughout the day. The juice is at its best fresh out of the juicer, but if you have a good masticating juicer your drink can last for up to twenty-four hours.

How do I keep it fresh?
Heat, air, and light destroy the juice. If you're making a quart of juice in the morning and want to keep it fresh all day, here is the best procedure to follow:

Take an opaque flask and remove the cap.
Put the flask in the freezer for the 15–30 minutes it takes you to juice your fruit and veggies. Once you're done, get the flask out of the freezer and pour the juice in.
Add ice to keep it cold all day.
This flask trick will make sure your juice stays free of heat, air, and light and keep it fresher for longer.

Getting ready to start
The very first step is of course to buy a good-quality masticating juicer such as the Oscar. (For more information on juicers, which one to buy and where to buy one, turn to page 36 in Our Raw Food Kitchen or page 219 for Resources).

Get set, go!
Now that you are ready to reap the health benefits of juicing, let's begin.
The best way to start is by juicing the vegetables you'd normally enjoy eating.
The following guidelines and recipes will help take the guesswork out of juicing. The basic rule is to start with a sweet base while you learn to like the taste of the greens. If the juice is too strong in the early stages and you don't enjoy it, you won't stick to it, so ease yourself in gently.

How to enhance your juice:
The question you should always be asking yourself in relation to nutrition is:
How can I enhance the nutrient density of the meal I am having so that I can get even more goodness into my body?

The easiest way to do this is to add superfood powders to your juices. There are many to choose from. The following combine well with green juices.

Powdered Greens such as:
Barleygrass and wheatgrass powders
These are highly concentrated forms of grasses providing unmatched mineral density.

Algae such as:
Blue-green algae, spirulina powder, and chlorella
Algae powders are the highest protein foods on the planet, at approximately 60 percent protein by weight. They provide high-quality, complete protein.

MSM
MSM is an organic form of sulfur that aids digestion by increasing nutrient absorption. MSM stimulates good hair and nail growth and glowing skin. It has also been found to be an essential nutrient for bone and joint health.

Step 1: Start Simple

Basically Green

Makes 1 generous cup (250–300 mL),
dilute with the same quantity of water to make 2 cups (500–600 mL)

2 apples
½ cucumber
2 celery stalks
½ lemon

Juice all the ingredients and dilute with water.

Apples combine well with vegetable juices, making them sweeter and more palatable. Apples, cucumber, and celery are light and gentle on the digestive system. Cucumber is a good source of potassium and celery is an excellent source of sodium. The celery leaves make the juice taste a little bitter, so remove them if you find the taste of the leaves overwhelming.

Easy-drinking Green

Makes 1 generous cup (250–300 mL),
dilute with the same quantity of water to make 2 cups (500–600 mL)

1 apple
1–2 carrots
½ cucumber
2 celery stalks
½ pineapple

Juice all the ingredients and dilute with water.

Another easy-drinking mild green juice, this includes a base of pineapple and carrots, which are naturally sweet. Let the pineapple, carrots, and apple make up approximately half of the total volume of juice.

The natural organic sodium in celery is essential for the body. Celery is known to contain at least eight families of anti-cancer compounds, and has been shown to effectively and significantly lower cholesterol.

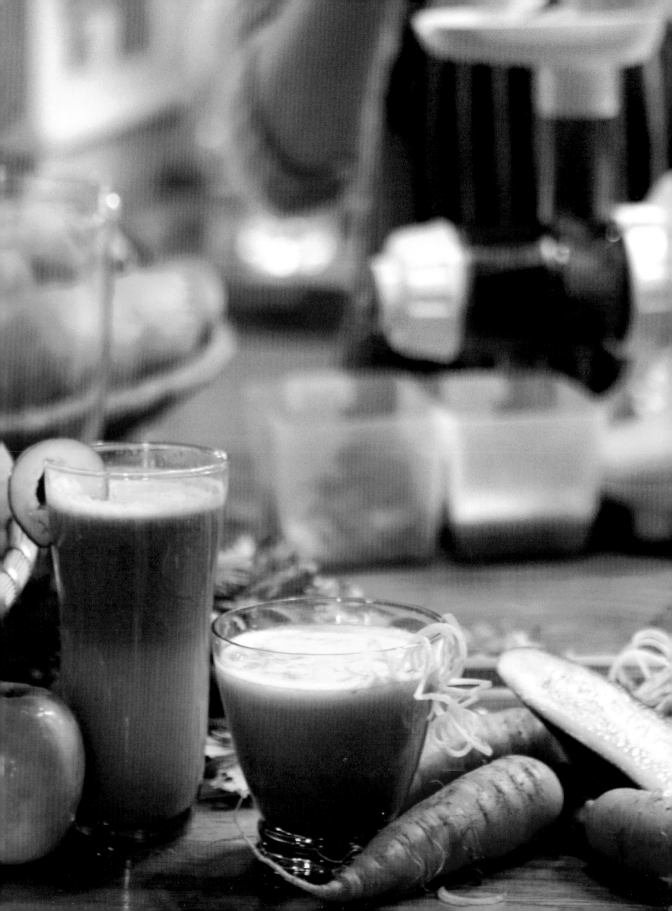

Step 2: Begin to Add Darker Green Leaves

Once you've gotten used to the simple veggie juices, make them more nutritionally dense by adding some of the following:

Getting Stronger

Makes 1 generous cup (250–300 mL),
dilute with the same quantity of water to make 2 generous cups (500–600 mL)

1 apple
½ cucumber
2 carrots
2 celery stalks
1 handful red or green lettuce leaves
1 handful spinach or swiss chard
2 bok choi leaves
5 tatsoi leaves

Juice all the ingredients
and dilute with water.

Green leaves are important to add to your juice. They are packed with enzymes and magnesium and are very alkalizing to the body.

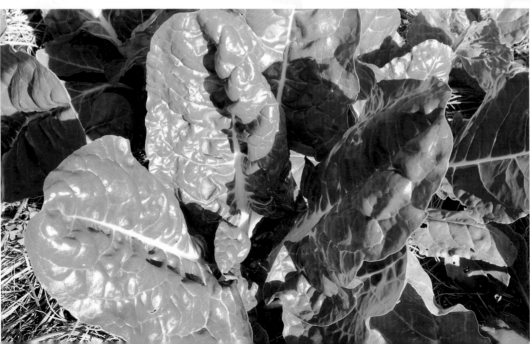

The Secret Ingredient

Lemon is a non-sweet fruit and, surprisingly enough, is alkalizing to the body and aids digestion.

Secrets Revealed

Makes 2 generous cups (500–750 mL),
dilute with the same quantity of water to make 4
generous cups (1–1 ½ liters)

2 apples
1 grapefruit
1 cucumber
½ bunch of celery
5 big leaves spinach or swiss chard
3 big leaves kale
1 lemon

Juice all the ingredients and dilute with water.

Do yourself a favor and begin adding lemon to your juice. Adding lemon to your green vegetable juices makes the juice refreshing and at the same time hides the taste of the stronger dark-green leaves. If your lemons are organic you can juice them with the peel. There is a lot of goodness in the pith.

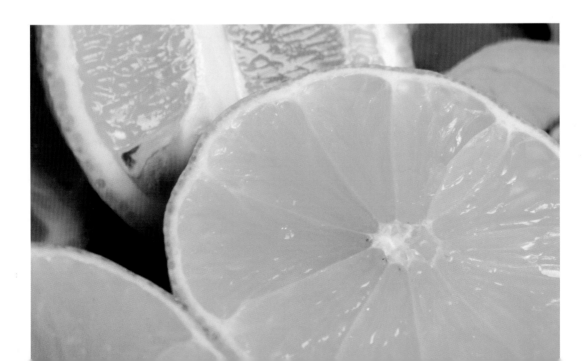

Step 3: Putting it All Together

The Green Alkalizer

Makes 2 cups (500 mL),
dilute with the same quantity of water to make 4 cups (1 liter)

This is the green juice we start our days off with.

1 apple
½ grapefruit or orange
½ cucumber
½ lemon
5 celery stalks
4 spinach leaves
1 sprig parsley
1 segment of fennel
1 kale leaf
2 bok choi leaves
3 tatsoi leaves

Juice all the ingredients and dilute with water.

If you are drinking a quart or more of this juice per day, it can probably take the place of a meal. At the very least it will discourage mid-morning and mid-afternoon snacking.

The Green Alkalizer is where the real nutrition is at. This juice is loaded with enzymes, antioxidants, magnesium, potassium, sodium, vitamins, and minerals. It is cleansing and alkalizing and is packed with living water. A juice like this can also help to keep blood-sugar levels stable.

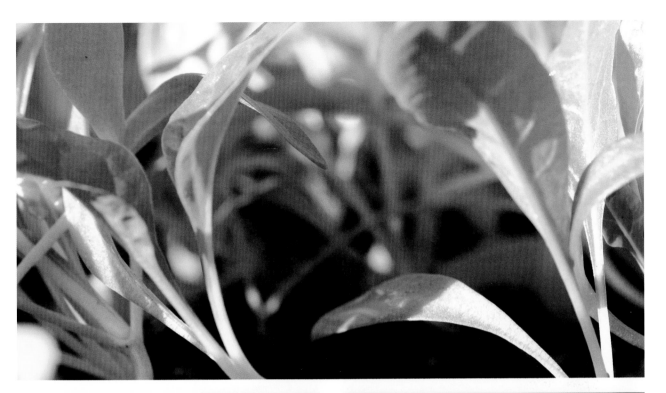

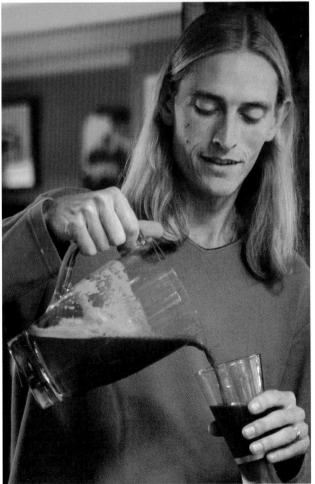

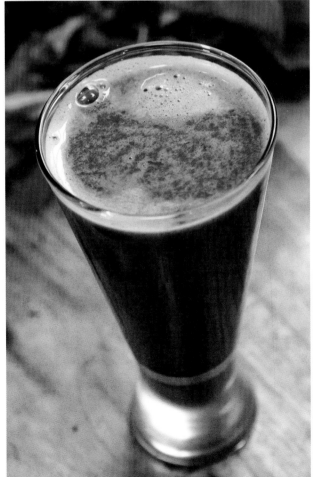

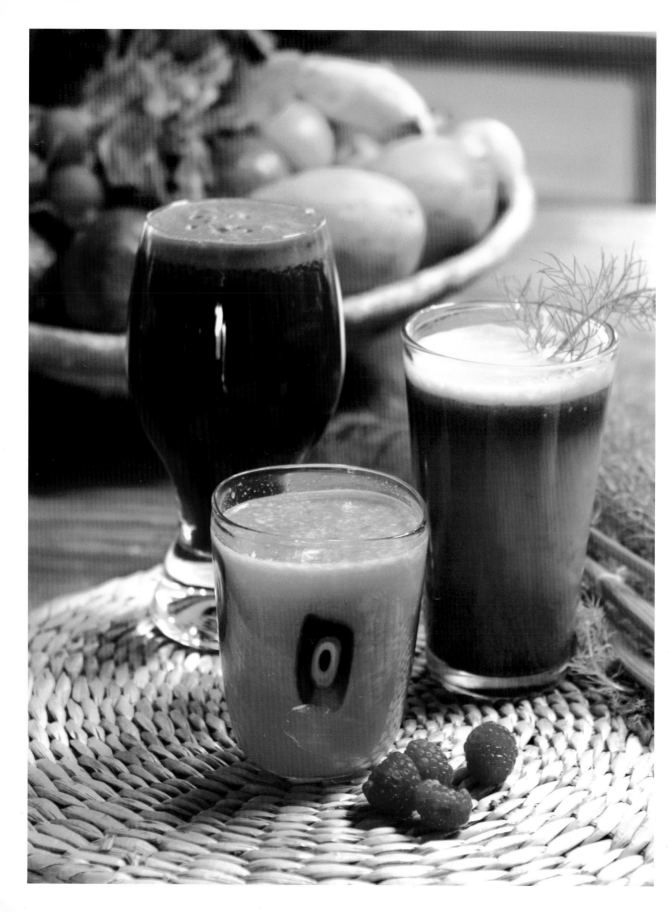

Have Some Fun

Get creative; turn your green juice red, purple, or brown! Add raw beet for a great variation in color and taste. It's also cleansing for the liver and the blood. Remember that adding beet to very dark greens can make the juice a muddy brown color.

Red Red Wine

Makes 1 cup (250 mL), undiluted

2 apples
½ cucumber
2 beets

Juice all the ingredients together and pour into wine glasses.

Green Cocktail

Makes 1 cup (250 mL), undiluted

2 apples
½ cucumber
1 medium fennel bulb

Juice all the ingredients.

This cocktail is so delicious; you can even serve it to your friends.

Fruity Sunrise

Makes 2 cups (500 mL), undiluted

½ pineapple
2 oranges
1 handful of strawberries or raspberries
1 wedge lemon

Juice all the ingredients.

Foraging in Your Garden

Makes 1 cup (250 mL), undiluted

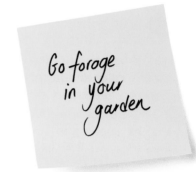

1 cucumber
1 apple
1 lemon
1 handful wild greens

Wild Greens:
stinging nettles – uncommon in South Africa but mild and delicious if you can find them
dandelion greens – these are lawn weeds!
sorrel - small to large leaves with a spear-like shape and a delicious, lemony flavor
nasturtiums – peppery round leaves, very common in winter
clovers – grow everywhere, delicious tart taste

Juice all the ingredients.

Learning which of the wild plants in your garden are edible is one of the most rewarding things you can do. You can increase the nutrient density of your juice for free by foraging in your garden for wild greens.

The surprising thing about stinging nettles is that when you drink them, they *don't sting!* Your saliva neutralizes all the stingers.
Stinging nettle tip: Use gloves when collecting stinging nettle.

Wild greens are loaded with up to fifty times more minerals than conventionally grown produce because they come from unfarmed soils.

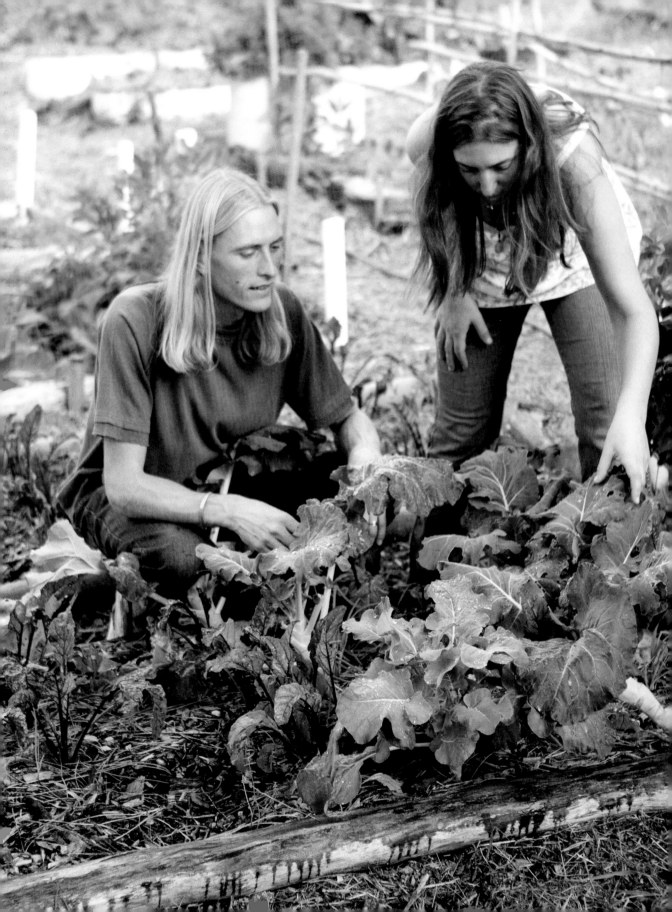

Go Back to Bed

Try adding ginger, garlic, and fennel when you're feeling a bit under the weather. All of these are nature's antibiotics. Dose up on this juice, get into bed, and you'll be bouncing around again in no time at all.

Time for Some Rest

Makes 2 cups (500 mL), undiluted

½ pineapple
1 orange
1 lemon
2 carrots
1 large clove garlic
Approx. 1 inch (2 cm) piece ginger
½ fennel bulb

Juice all the ingredients.

P.S. It's better to steer clear of your friends when drinking this one.

Ginger, garlic, and fennel are nature's antibiotics.

Spice It Up

Makes 2 cups (500 mL), undiluted

2 clementines
1 grapefruit
½ lemon
½ inch (1 cm) piece ginger
1 wedge aloe ferox or aloe vera

Cut a 2 inch (5 cm) wedge of aloe ferox/vera, remove the skin from the inner gel and rinse away any yellow bitters. Juice all the ingredients.

Cut & rinse your wedge of aloe first

Radically Radish

Makes 2 cups (500 mL), undiluted

2 grapefruit
5 radishes
1 pear

Juice all the ingredients.

The radishes in this juice give it a spicy kick. Combined with the grapefruit, they make for a great liver-support juice. This juice is also called the Potent Pink Juice because of its phenomenal color.

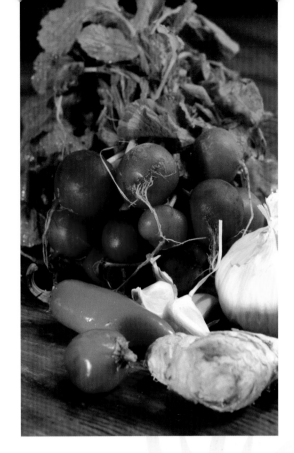

Apple-chili Cleanser

Makes 2 cups (500 mL), undiluted

2 apples
½ cucumber
¼ lemon
½ inch (1 cm) piece ginger
1 pinch cayenne pepper

Juice all the ingredients.

This juice is delicious and the flecks of cayenne pepper make a refreshing variation on the normal green juice look. Beyond aesthetics, cayenne pepper has many other benefits.

Chilis are loaded with vitamin C and their stimulating properties power more nutrition into your cells.

A Touch of Garnish

Adding certain herbs to your juices facilitates cleansing and detoxification.

Rich & Creamy

Makes 1 generous cup (250–300 mL), undiluted

2 apples
2 pears
1 small handful grapes
1 small handful parsley
1 wedge lemon

Juice all the ingredients.

*Parsley
is a great source of
minerals, especially iro
Aloe ferox, or aloe ver
is one of the top wild
superfoods and is the b
source of glyconutrien
– essential sugars for
cellular heath.*

Therapeutic Juicing

There are a variety of herbs, sprouts, and grasses that are vital to a therapeutic juicing regime. They are medicinal, so be warned – you may not like the taste to begin with.

These juices are best consumed on their own and knocked back in a single shot glass (30 mL).

The Cilantro Cure

Makes 1 cup (250 mL), undiluted

½ apple
¼ cucumber
1 wedge lemon
1 handful cilantro

Juice all the ingredients.

*Cilantro is excellent for
detoxifying heavy metals from
the body. It is especially good
at binding the mercury from
amalgam dental fillings and
flushing it out of the body.*

A Shot of Grass

Makes 5 shot glasses (5 x 30 mL)

1 tray wheatgrass

Cut the grass just above the soil and juice using a masticating juicer.
(A centrifugal juicer will not juice wheatgrass.)

It is best to drink your wheatgrass as soon as it has been juiced
for maximum potency.

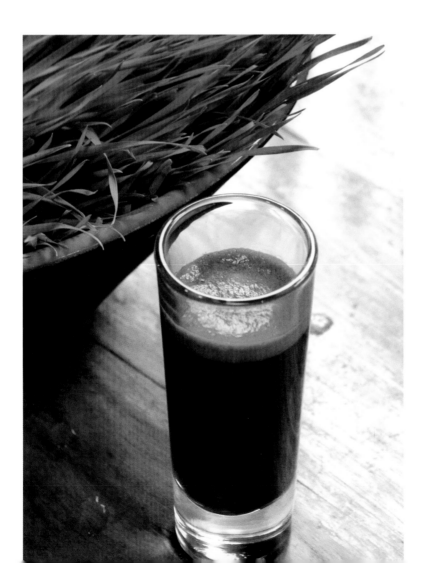

The Grass Is Greener

It is said that one shot of wheatgrass is equivalent to two plates of vegetables.

Makes 1 cup (250 mL),
dilute with the same quantity of water to make 2 cups (500 mL)

1 apple
½ lemon
1 tray wheatgrass

Juice all the ingredients.

The grass really is greener on the other side of this drink. While many people find straight wheatgrass quite hard to stomach, most find this version much more palatable. As I've already mentioned, the health benefits of juicing wheatgrass are enormous. It's incredibly detoxifying, so power up to wheatgrass slowly. Let your body get used to the alkalizing effects of green juicing with the simpler recipes first. Then move on to this king of the greens.

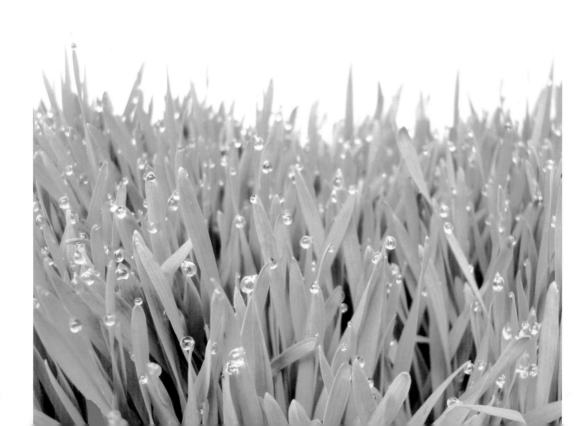

Sunflower Sprout Health

Makes 1 cup (250 mL),
dilute with the same quantity of water to make
2 cups (500 mL)

1 apple
1 carrot
½ tray sunflower sprouts

Add ½ tray of wheatgrass to this concoction
to elevate it to supreme health-juice status!

Juice all the ingredients.

Another simple green to grow at home is sunflower greens. They are grown in the same way as wheatgrass. Surprisingly enough, mixing sunflower greens with wheatgrass, apple, and carrot makes the entire concoction rather tasty.

Grow your own microgreens

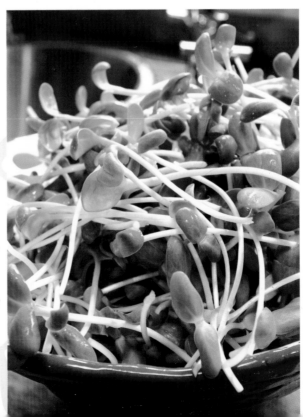

Sunflower greens are around ten times more nutritious than lettuce. In fact, the combination of wheatgrass and sunflower greens is key to all therapeutic juicing protocols.

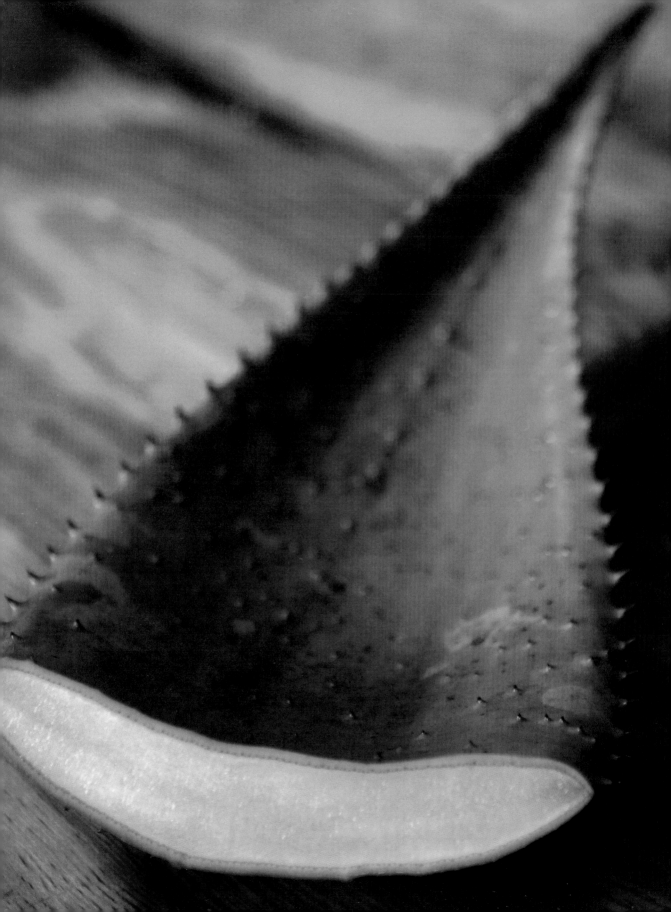

Cleansing Classics

The Cape Classic

Makes 3 cups (750 mL)

2 cups (500 mL) water
½ aloe leaf
3 apples
Approx ½ inch (1 cm) piece ginger
1 lemon
1 sprig fresh buchu or mint

Juice all the ingredients.

This is a fantastic detox juice.
We've called it the Cape Classic
because it combines two of the Western
Cape's great superfoods.

Aloe ferox or aloe vera stimulates the production of collagen in the body, which maintains flexibility in the skin, bones, joints, and tissues. Buchu is known as a "heal-all" herb and has been used traditionally to treat all manner of ailments. It is an overall immune-boosting tonic and diuretic.

Mint-apple-aloe Cooler

Makes 1 small cup (200 mL) undiluted
Dilute with 7 tablespoons (100 mL) water for a glass (300 mL)

2 apples
1 wedge aloe
1 handful fresh mint

Juice all the ingredients.

This one is a big favorite in our household
because it is so simple and refreshing.

Using Aloe Ferox or Aloe Vera

Aloe ferox and aloe vera make wonderful additions to juices and smoothies. They are widely available in nurseries, so be sure to plant them in your garden. The leaves have sharp thorns along the edges and angle towards the sky.

The best leaves to pick are the lower ones that are about to turn brown and become the dried leaves around the stem. If you pick the top leaves you will be killing the plant. The leaves are ripe when the tips have a slightly red blush.

Don't overpick from one aloe plant and don't pick from baby aloes.

To pick the leaf you need a sharp knife and a bag. Cut as close to the stem as possible. A bright yellow liquid will run out of the cut leaf; these are the aloe bitters.

This is how you harvest and prepare aloe ferox and aloe vera.

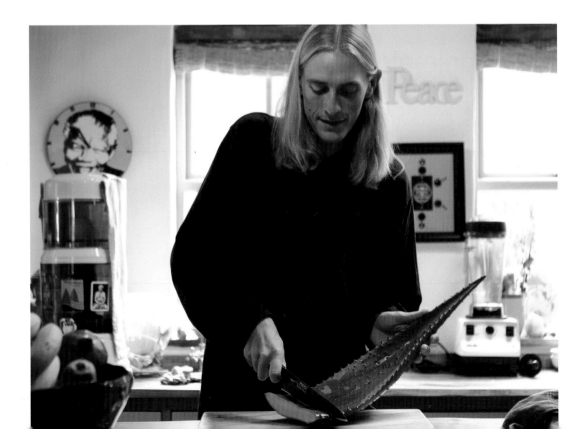

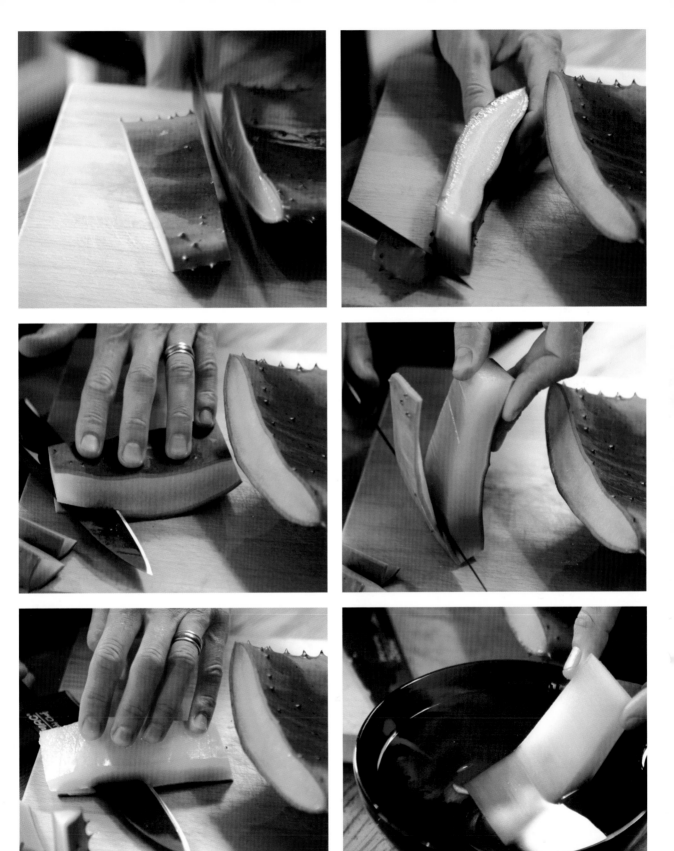

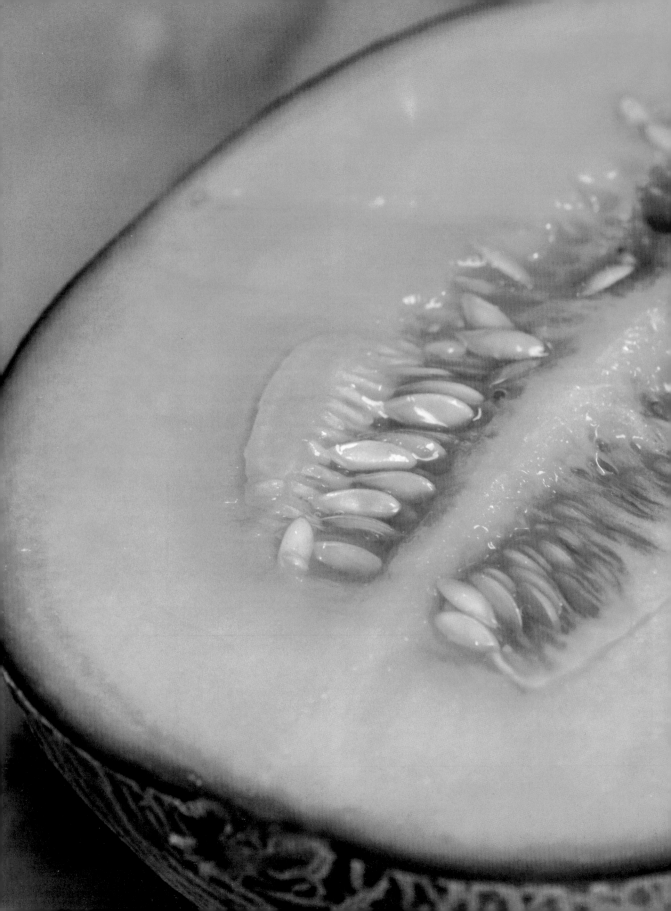

Smoothies

The Blender Chef

One of easiest ways to get into eating more raw foods without having to get your head around the gourmet stuff is to become a blender chef.

If you are one of those people who simply doesn't like spending time in the kitchen slaving over a hot stove, then blending is a quick, easy, and delicious way to get great food in without all the fuss.

At home, Peter is our blender chef. The Vitamix is his favorite alchemical tool. Being a blender chef is all about having fun, playing and experimenting with mixing up a variety of different ingredients into new and interesting combinations.

The best place to start is with smoothies.

The Ingredients

Water
The best base for your smoothie is not some white liquid from another mammal. It is high-quality spring water.

Soft fruit
Bananas are the best fruit for sweetening and thickening your smoothie, but mangos and berries make delicious alternatives.

Nuts
Almonds and brazil nuts tend to work best and taste the nicest.

Natural sweeteners
Use honey, dates, or agave to sweeten your smoothies naturally.

Superfoods
There is a wide array of superfoods you can choose from to boost your smoothies. Our favorites are goji berries, raw cacao, green powders, and maca powder.

Add some ice to make sure your smoothies stay cold or, for extra thickness, use peeled frozen bananas instead.

In our kitchen we don't use recipes for smoothies. Instead, we have large baskets of fruit on the counter and all our superfoods are kept on a shelf in glass jars. Every morning, Peter will pick whichever ingredients catch his eye and whip up something new and tasty. If you get into the habit of starting your day off with a green vegetable juice and some kind of superfood smoothie you will most likely be getting in more nutrition than the average person on a "normal" diet gets in a week!

But blending isn't only limited to smoothies. You can also make soups, pestos, pâtés, sauces, and even nut butters using a high-power blender. Eating and drinking blended foods is probably our favorite way of eating. Sometimes we will go the whole day just on liquid foods and feel completely satisfied, satiated, and energized at the end of the day. The best thing about adopting the blending approach is that you spend no more than fifteen minutes in the kitchen per meal.

We have found that most people already own some kind of blending device. You don't have to have fancy, expensive blending equipment to get started. A simple, hand-held stick blender can suffice. Ultimately you'll want to equip your kitchen with a high-speed power blender, though.

As with all the recipes in this book, these are a guideline and an outline of how to bridge the gap between where you are now and where you would like to be. We hope these recipes will serve as a springboard from which to launch into your own new world of smoothie magic.

Remember to have fun and play with your food.

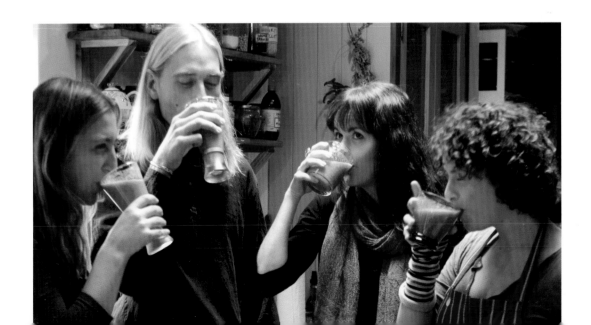

Melon Cream

Serves 2–3

This is the simplest smoothie I make and you'll be surprised at how creamy and delicious it is. The key lies in adding the seeds, which contain good oils and have anti-parasitic properties.

1 honeydew melon with seeds
1 teaspoon camu camu berry powder (optional)

Scoop the melon and the seeds into your blender. Blend until smooth.

As melons digest very quickly, they should usually be eaten on their own with no other ingredients added. However, camu camu berry powder is one of the few superfoods that mixes really well with melon and gives it a slight zing.

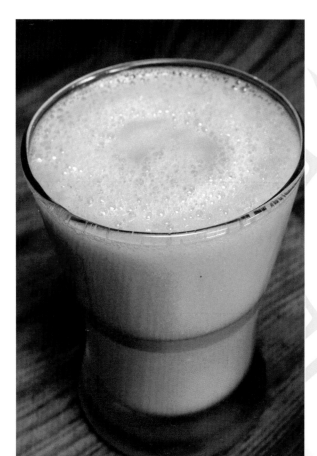

Camu camu berries come from the Amazon and are the highest-known source of vitamin C. Melons are also a good source of vitamin C and potassium.

Super-berry Milkshake

Serves 2–3

Prepare almond milk first

I normally indulge in this one during those few short weeks when organic strawberries are in season. It is scrumptious.

1 cup (250 mL) almond milk (see page 78)
1 large banana
1 tablespoon honey
5 Brazil nuts
1 large handful strawberries, raspberries, blackberries, blueberries, or mulberries
1 pinch Himalayan rock salt
⅛ cup goji berries, soaked for 10 minutes (optional)

Make up a batch of almond milk (see page 78).
Put all the ingredients into a blender and blend until smooth.
Pour into glasses and enjoy.

Strawberries are one of the most pesticide-sprayed fruit crops, so when I can't get organic, I go for other berries such as blackberries, raspberries, mulberries, or blueberries.

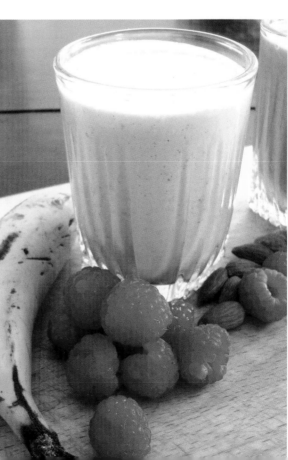

Joshua's Berry Berry Nice Smoothie

Serves 2–3

Joshua is one of my best friends in the whole wide world. At the time of this writing, he is almost six years old. I recently visited him and his family in London and was determined to get some green juice into him. Here's the smoothie we came up with together. Joshua drank it and declared it to be berry berry nice.

2–3 handfuls mixed berries such as blueberries, blackberries, raspberries, or strawberries
1 banana
1½ cups (375 mL) green juice (we used a mixture of cucumber, apple, carrot, and spinach)
2 teaspoons honey

Blend everything together.

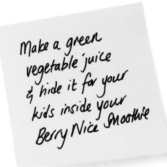

Make a green vegetable juice & hide it for your kids inside your Berry Nice Smoothie

Summer Cooler

Serves 4–6

1 watermelon
1 large handful mint

Scoop out the watermelon flesh and some of the seeds.
Blend with the mint.

Chocolate Smoothie

Serves 2

This is every chocaholic's dream – a perfectly raw, healthy, guilt-free chocolate "milkshake" for breakfast.

2 cups (500 mL) prepared almond or Brazil nut milk (see page 78 and 79)
1 banana
2 tablespoons honey
3 tablespoons cacao powder
2–4 tablespoons cacao nibs
1 teaspoon maca

Put all the ingredients into a power blender, keeping back 2 tablespoons cacao nibs if you want to add them in at the end for the chocolate-chip crunch. Blend all the ingredients until smooth. Stir in the extra 2 tablespoons cacao nibs and serve.

Cacao beans are a great source of magnesium and are second only to blue-green algae as the best antioxidant food in the world!

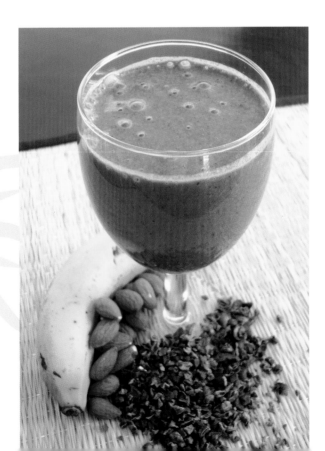

Aloe Citrus

Serves 3

Here we once again have the Cape's superfood ingredients – aloe ferox or aloe vera and buchu. Peter, Lexi, and I detoxed by drinking around 3 cups (750 mL) of this drink every day for three days while spending the rest of our time in the hot springs in Kwazulu-Natal.

2 grapefruit, juiced
2 oranges
2 inches (5 cm) wedge fresh aloe ferox or aloe vera
1 handful dried rosehips or 1 teaspoon camu camu berry powder
1 handful goji berries
1 sprig fresh buchu or mint
Approx ½ inch (1 cm) ginger
2 tablespoons honey
4 cups (1 liter) water
1 passion fruit (optional)
3 dried figs (optional)

Blend all the ingredients together in a blender.

The vitamin C level of this drink is off the charts. The aloe ferox or aloe vera is excellent for the digestive system and is also an anti-parasitic food.

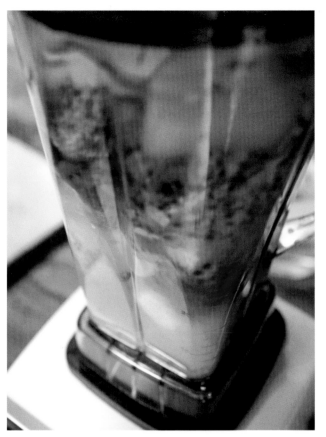
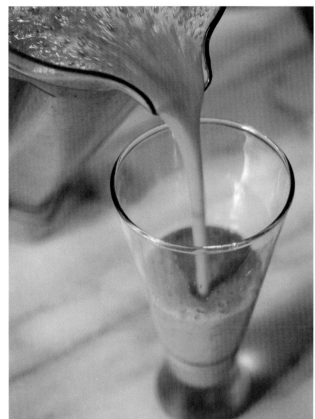
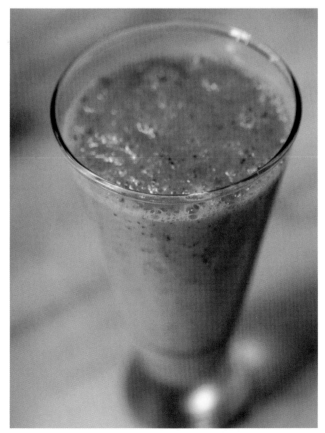
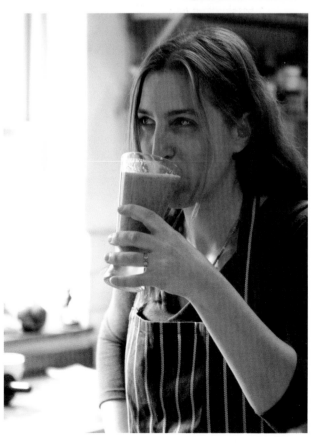

Green Smoothie

I first heard of the green smoothie concept in a short DVD by Victoria Boutenko. She and her entire family went raw overnight after they all came down with various life-threatening diseases in the same year. Getting a wide variety of green leaves into the diet is essential if you are going to succeed with a raw lifestyle. Making green smoothies was one of their tricks for getting in high volumes of greens easily. We've experimented with many different varieties. These are our favorites:

Option 1

Serves 2

1 cup (250 mL) water
1 banana
1 kiwi fruit
1 cup tightly packed spinach
5 pitted dates or dried figs
½–1 tablespoon honey, depending on your taste for sweetness

Blend and serve.

Option 2

Serves 2

1 cup (250 mL) water
½ pineapple
1 small lemon
1 cup tightly packed mixed green leaves
1 sprig mint or buchu

Blend and serve.

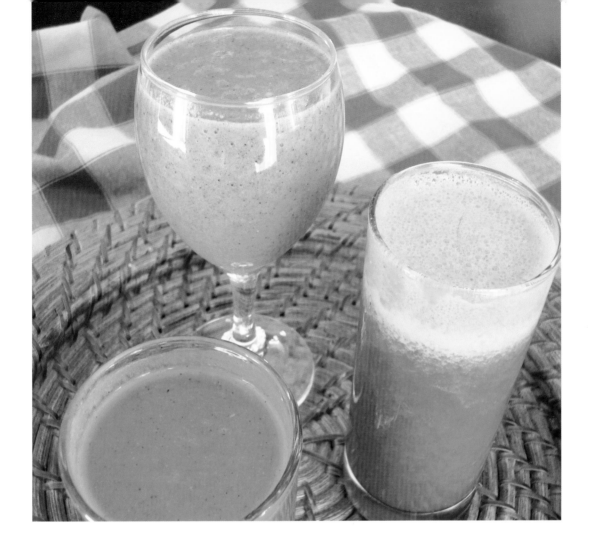

Blue-green Smoothie

Serves 2

1 cup (250 mL) water
2 kiwi fruit
1 banana
1 teaspoon honey
1 tablespoon blue-green algae or spirulina

Blend all the ingredients together, pour into glasses, and enjoy.

Maca Love

Serves 2

Maca has many claims to fame but is most famous as a natural aphrodisiac, hence the name of this recipe – Maca Love.
It has a slightly malty flavor and this smoothie comes out with a rich, almost Horlicks (malted milk) taste. It's a big favorite in our liquid elixirs class.

2 cups (500 mL) Brazil nut milk (see page 79)
5 pitted dates
2 figs
1 tablespoon maca
1 pinch Himalayan rock salt

Make a batch of Brazil nut milk (see page 79).
Combine all of the above ingredients and blend.

The Two-tone Sunrise

Serves 4

This one is a real feast for the eyes as well as for the stomach and is absolutely gorgeous as a summer sundowner when mangos are in season.

2 cups (500 mL) water
2 mangos
1 handful dried peaches
½ beet
1 orange

Blend the water, mangos, and dried peaches in a power blender until smooth and pour into glasses. Juice the beet and orange and pour over the mango.

Spiral Green

Serves 4–5

This one is affectionately known in our home as "the swamp." I am not a huge fan of the taste of spirulina and normally turn my nose up at any of Peter or Lexi's spirulina concoctions. However, Lexi made this drink one morning and brought it to me to taste and I couldn't believe it – it tasted great!

4 cups (1 liter) water
2 frozen bananas
1 mango
½ pineapple
1 tablespoon spirulina
1 teaspoon buchu powder or sprig of fresh mint
2 teaspoons hemp oil (optional)

Blend all the ingredients together and serve.

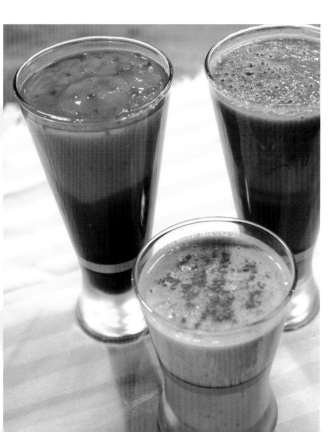

Spirulina contains 334% more protein than beef, 475% more calcium than whole milk, 5756% more iron than spinach, and is a rich source of B-complex vitamins, containing 118% more B12 than raw beef liver!

Superfood Smoothie

This Superfood Smoothie can sustain me for the entire day. This is the recipe that we teach on our two-day Raw Food Course. It has a simple superfood base of bananas, almond milk, and dates or honey, and then we add all the superfoods we can get our hands on.

This smoothie has so much nutritional goodness packed into it that if I have a glass at 10 a.m. I won't need to eat again until 3 p.m. or even 4 p.m.

4 cups (1 liter) water or 2 cups ice and 2 cups (500 mL) water
1 cup (250 mL) almond milk (see page 78)
1 large banana (frozen for cold milkshake)
3 tablespoons honey / agave / maple syrup / pitted dates to sweeten
½ teaspoon ground cinnamon
1 vanilla pod
5 brazil nuts
1 tablespoon hemp protein powder
1 handful goji berries
1 tablespoon maca powder
1 tablespoon green powder
3 tablespoons raw cacao powder / beans / nibs
1 pinch Himalayan rock salt
1 inch (2½ cm) wedge fresh aloe ferox or aloe vera
1–2 tablespoons coconut oil

Blend everything in a blender. Pour into a flask and enjoy throughout the day.

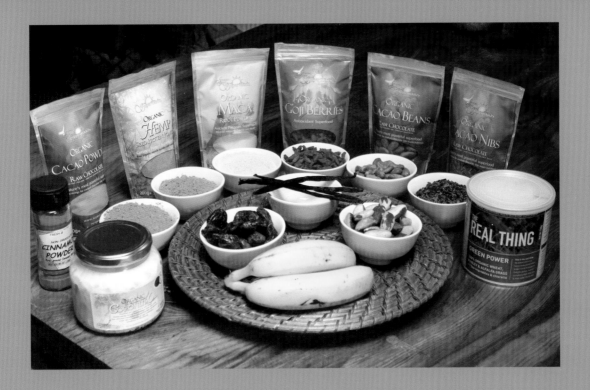

Aloe ferox/vera	excellent overall detoxifier
Raw honey	rich in enzymes
Cinnamon	helps to stabilize blood sugar levels
Brazil nuts	high in the mineral selenium
Hemp powder	a source of vegan protein containing all the essential amino acids
Goji berries	very high in vitamin C and antioxidants
Maca powder	a hormone-balancing food, strength builder, and natural aphrodisiac
Green powder	good for cleansing, detoxifying, and alkalizing
Raw cacao	great source of magnesium and a good-mood brain food
Himalayan salt	mineral-rich salt
Coconut oil	good plant-saturated fat that assists in lowering cholesterol and balancing hormones

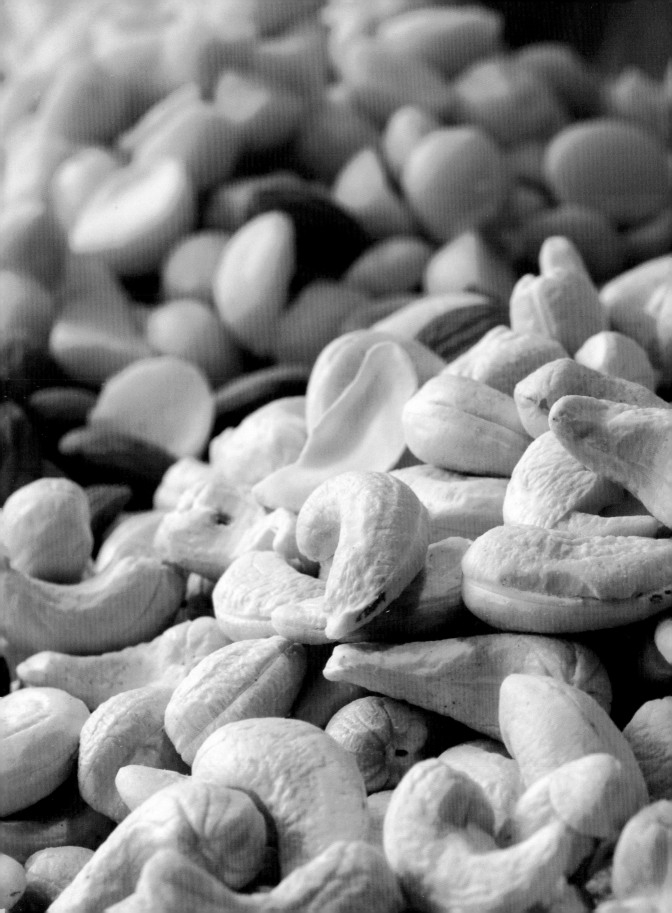

Nut Milks, Butters & Cheese

Almond Milk

Brazil Nut Milk

Sesame Milk

Chocolate Milk

Macadamia Nut Butter

Cashew Nut Butter

Brazil Nut Butter

Instant Cashew Nut Cheese

Cream Cheese

How to Make Nut Milks

Once you've tasted nut milk, ditching dairy is an easy task. Making nut milk is very quick and easy, and once you know how to make it you can use it in a variety of recipes to replace all sorts of dairy products. You can use it in smoothies to replace milk or yoghurt, you can pour it over your breakfast cereal, and you can even use it to make ice cream. The pulp can also be dried, stored, and used later in other recipes.

1. Blend the nuts and water.
2. Strain through a nut milk bag or strainer.
3. Pour the milk into a glass jar and store.
4. Turn the nut pulp out onto a solid dehydrator sheet and dehydrate until dry.
5. Put the dry pulp in a dry blender and powder into flour.
6. Store the flour in a glass jar for use in cookies later.

How to Make Nut Butters

You will need a power blender for this, and your blender will have to work quite hard to get the right consistency, but the effort is worth it, as a jar of raw nut butter in the refrigerator goes a long way. You simply put nuts into the blender without anything else and, using the tamper to make sure the blades are reaching everything, blend until a soft, smooth paste is formed.

How to Make Nut Cheese

Nut cheese is simply heavenly. We discovered this recipe completely by accident. I'd made up a batch of macadamia-based cream, put the jar in the refrigerator and forgot about it. A few days later, when I was clearing the refrigerator, I found the cream and nearly threw it out, assuming it would be off by then. But when I opened the jar, the mixture smelled just like cream cheese and when I tried it, it tasted just like cream cheese, too! Since then, we've perfected the fermentation process by adding probiotic cultures.

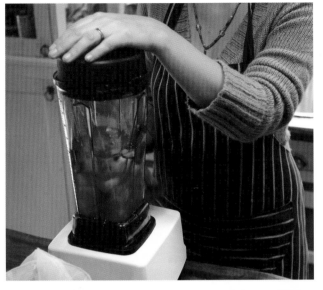
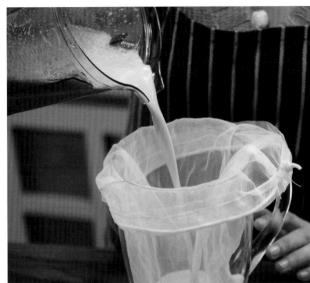
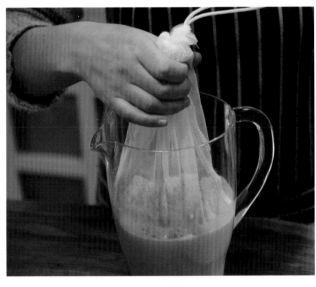
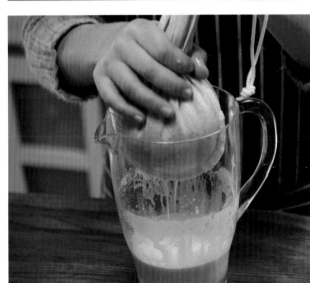
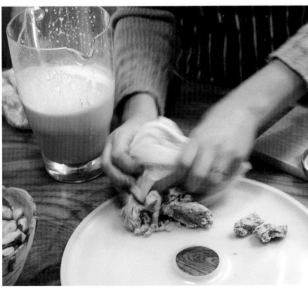
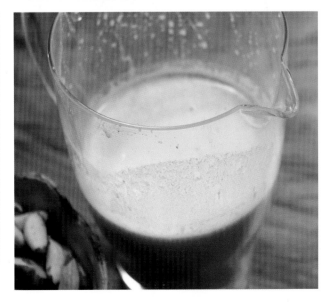

Nut Milks

Almond Milk

4 cups (1 liter) water
1 cup almonds, soaked and rinsed
5 dried figs or pitted dates
1 tablespoon honey
1 vanilla pod

Blend all the ingredients in a power blender and strain through a nut milk bag.

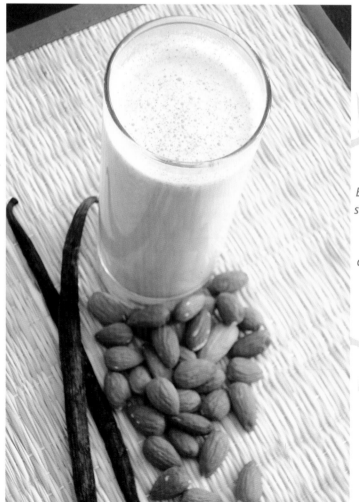

By soaking nuts and seeds, the digestion-straining enzyme inhibitors they contain are washed away and their life and vitality is increased.

Brazil Nut Milk

3 cups (750 mL) water
1 handful Brazil nuts
1 tablespoon honey
1 vanilla pod
2 dried figs

Blend all the ingredients in a power blender and strain through a nut milk bag.

Sesame Milk

3 cups (750 mL) water
1 cup sesame seeds
2 tablespoons honey

Blend all the ingredients in a power blender and strain through a nut milk bag.

Chocolate Milk

2 cups (500 mL) almond or Brazil nut milk
2 tablespoons honey
3 tablespoons cacao powder

Blend all the ingredients in a power blender.

Nut Butters

Macadamia Nut Butter

2–3 cups macadamia nuts

Cashew Nut Butter

2–3 cups cashews

Brazil Nut Butter

2–3 cups Brazil nuts

Blend the nuts in a high-speed blender such as the Vitamix for approximately 3 minutes on high speed, using the tamper to keep the mixture moving until a nut butter consistency is reached. 2–3 cups of nuts makes about 1 cup (200–300 mL) of nut butter. Your blender has to work really hard to get this one right, but a machine like the Vitamix can and does handle it.

See page 149 for my favorite nut butter snack.

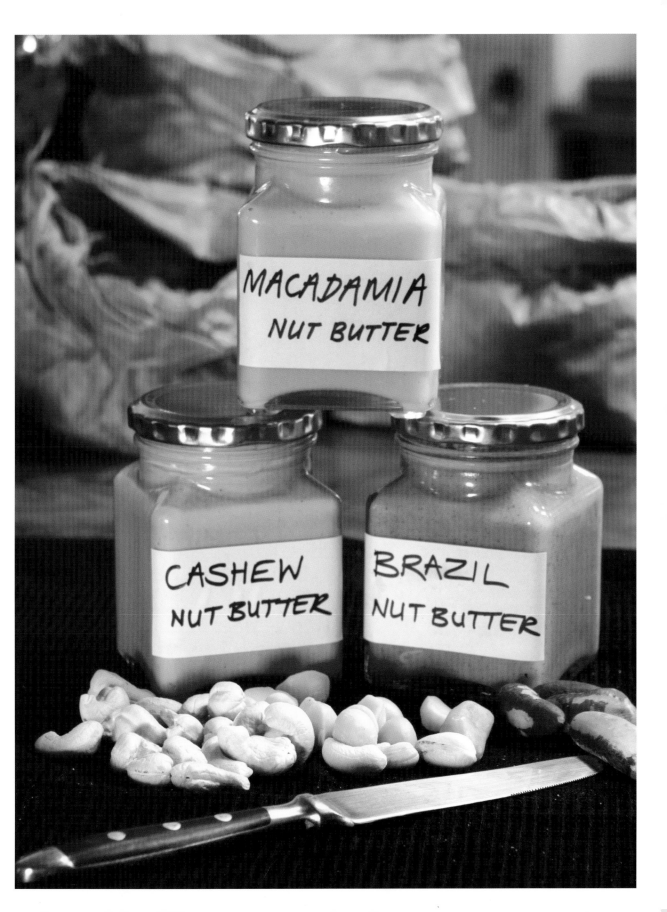

Nut Cheese

Instant Cashew Nut Cheese

Makes 1 quart

3 cups cashews
2 cups (500 mL) water
1 tablespoon nutritional yeast
⅛ small red onion
1 teaspoon agave
1 teaspoon Himalayan rock salt

Blend everything together in a power blender until completely smooth.

Cream Cheese

Makes 1 quart

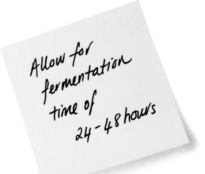

Allow for fermentation time of 24 - 48 hours

2½ cups macadamias
2 cups (500 mL) water
1 tablespoon lemon juice
1 tablespoon agave
1 teaspoon Himalayan rock salt
4 probiotic capsules

Blend all the ingredients except the probiotics together in a power blender until the nut cheese is completely smooth. Empty the contents of the probiotic capsules into the mix and blend through on low speed.

Divide the mixture into three jars of approx 1⅓ cups (300 mL) each.
Leave one jar plain and put it in the refrigerator.

Create other flavors such as:

Black Pepper Cream Cheese

1 teaspoon black peppercorns

Add 1 teaspoon black peppercorns and blend briefly.
Put in a jar and refrigerate.

Herb and Garlic

½ tablespoon mixed herbs
1 clove garlic

Add mixed herbs and garlic and blend briefly. Put in a jar and refrigerate.
Allow to ferment in the refrigerator for at least 24 hours and use within a week.

Experiment with other flavors such as cumin and cilantro or chili-flavored cream cheese.

Probiotics are powerful immunity boosters and are essential for proper digestion. They also predigest the nuts for better absorption.

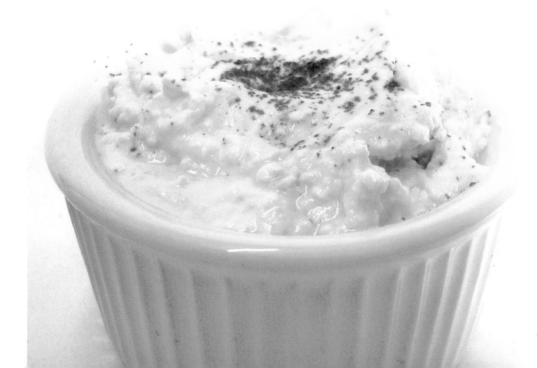

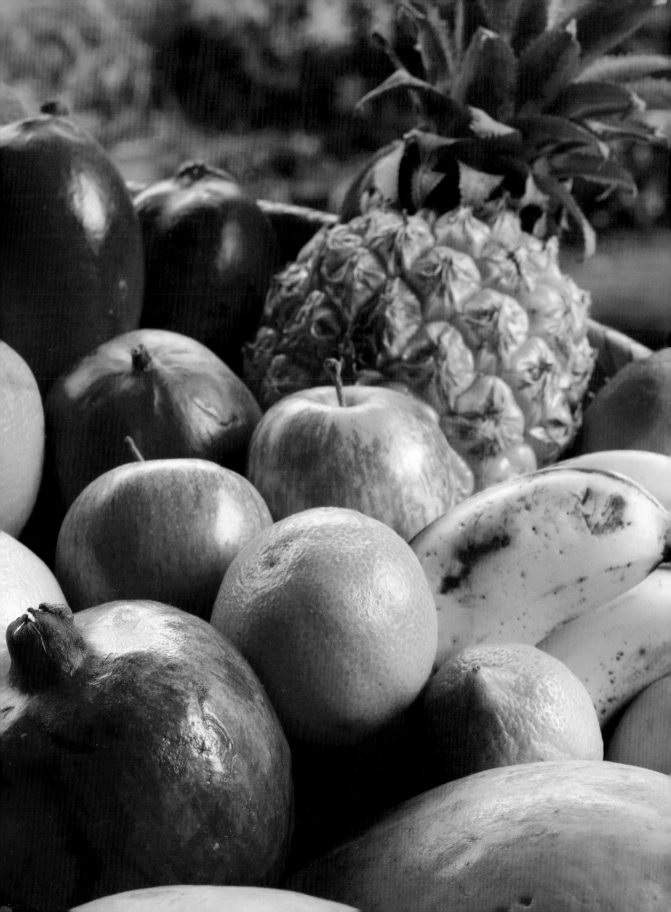

Breakfasts

If you feel like a bit of variation to the staple green vegetable juice and smoothie breakfast routine, give some of these other breakfast options a go.

Sweet Oatmeal

When you cook oats you make them very stodgy and difficult to digest. This is a much better way to prepare them. This recipe goes down very well with children.

uncooked rolled oats
apple juice
ground cinnamon
raisins
honey

Take 1 portion of rolled oats and place in a bowl. Don't use quick-cook oats as these have been precooked.
Juice your apples, pour the juice over the oats, and leave to soak overnight in the refrigerator. In the morning you will have delicious, sweet oatmeal.

Top with raisins, cinnamon, and honey.

The complex carbs in oats allow for a slower release of blood sugars, and oats are safe for those who are gluten intolerant.

Simple Buckwheat Cereal

Serve with almond milk (see page 78)

Serve with almond milk (see page 78)

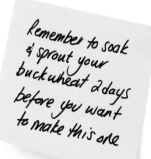

Remember to soak & sprout your buckwheat 2 days before you want to make this one

This is a simple recipe for buckwheat cereal, which stores very well in a glass jar. You can make up a batch on the weekend and store it for 1–2 weeks.

18 oz (500 g) hulled buckwheat, soaked and sprouted
3 tablespoons ground cinnamon
¾ cup honey
3 chopped apples

See page 24 for how to sprout buckwheat.
Mix the honey, cinnamon, and apples through the sprouted buckwheat. If the honey is too thick, thin it down with a little warm water. Spread the mixture out onto a solid dehydrator sheet. Place in the dehydrator and dehydrate for 24 hours. Store in a glass jar.

To serve, fill a breakfast bowl with buckwheat cereal and top with almond milk. You can also top this breakfast with freshly sliced banana and goji berries.

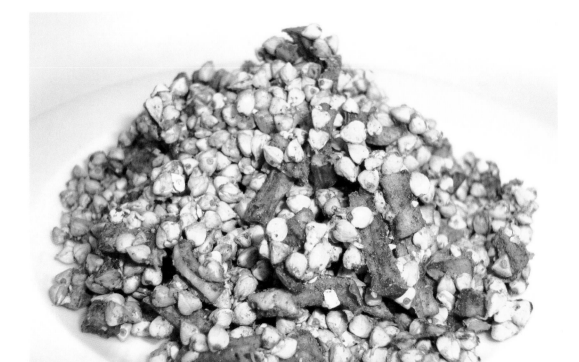

Breakfast Muesli

Enhance your simple buckwheat cereal with the following ingredients:

1 chopped pear
3 sliced bananas
½ cup almonds, soaked
1 cup sunflower seeds
1 cup goji berries
½ cup cacao nibs
½ cup raisins

Make up the Simple Buckwheat Cereal as in the previous recipe.
Pulse the almonds and sunflower seeds in a food processor until roughly chopped. Add to the cereal mix. Add in the remaining ingredients and mix through thoroughly. Place on dehydrator sheets and dehydrate until completely dry (approximately 24 hours).

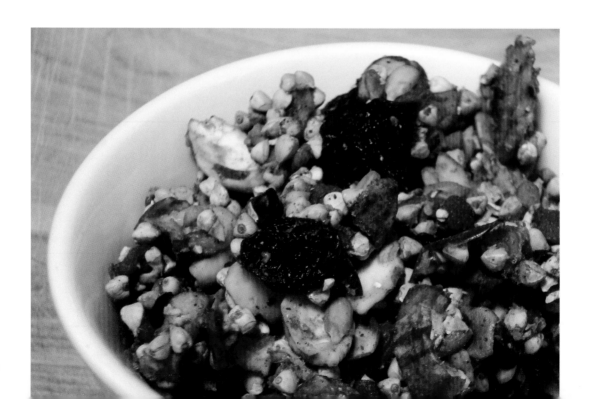

Fruit Sauce (or baby food)

I love this breakfast! It is fast to prepare and fun to make with children.

1 medium papaya
1 mango
1 banana

Blend all the ingredients in a blender or food processor.

Option 1: top with goji berries, passion fruit, Brazil nuts, and a swirl of sesame milk.

Option 2: Smiley face for children. Blend some dark berries such as raspberries or blueberries with a little water and use the mixture to draw a smiley face or write the first letter of your child's name on top of the sauce.

Remember to have fun and
play with your food.

*Papayas are
a rich source of proteolytic enzymes, which
enable the digestion of protein. The seeds are one of
nature's most powerful parasite remedies.*

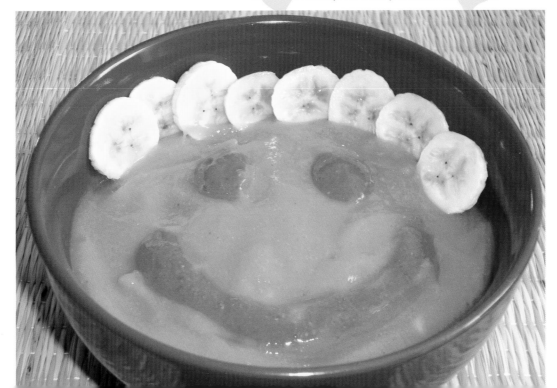

Nutty Fruit Salad with Maca Cream

Fruit salad is a wonderful, fresh way to start the day but I normally find that if I have only fruit salad for breakfast I am hungry again within two hours. However, when I add the maca cream, the combination of the maca and the nuts slows the release of the fruit sugars into the body so that the meal satiates me for longer.

A selection of seasonal fruit such as:
 papaya
 banana
 berries
 passion fruit
 pears
A selection of nuts and seeds:
 Brazil nuts
 macadamia nuts
 flaxseed (finely ground in a coffee grinder)
 pumpkin seeds
 sunflower seeds
A selection of superfoods:
 cacao nibs
 goji berries
 raw honey

Dice 2–3 different types of seasonal fresh fruit into a bowl.
Sprinkle with nuts, flaxseed, and sunflower and pumpkin seeds.
Top with goji berries and cacao nibs.
Drizzle with raw honey and enjoy.

Maca Cream

To make the maca cream, blend:

1 ½ cups (375 mL) water
1 cup macadamia nuts
1 tablespoon honey
1 teaspoon ground cinnamon
1 tablespoon maca powder

Adding maca to your breakfasts reduces your appetite.

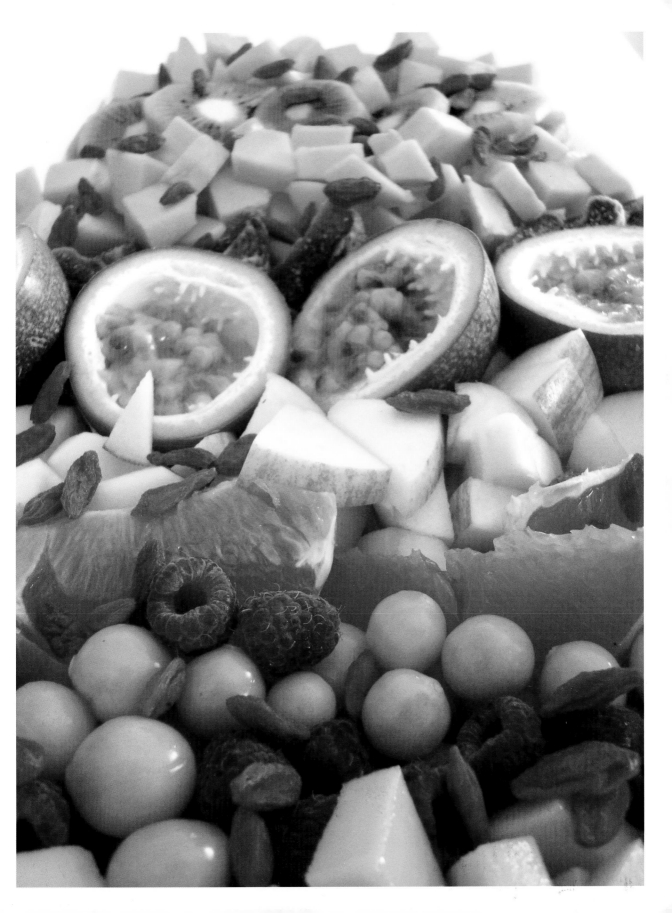

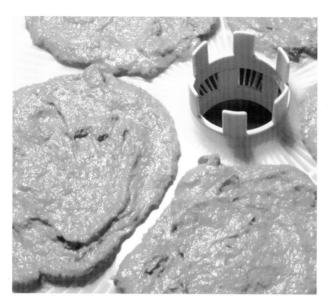

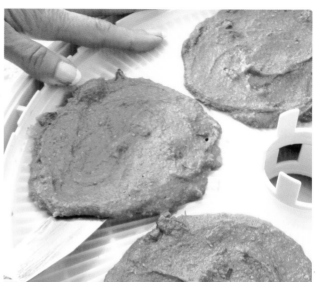

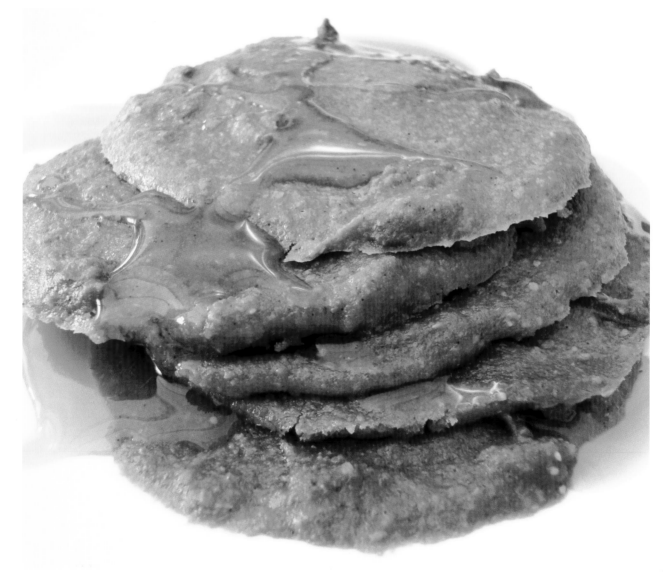

Pancakes

Makes 20–24 pancakes

This is a real Sunday morning treat.

½ cup goji berries, soaked and drained
2 bananas
2 cups pecans, soaked
½ cup pine nuts
½ cup golden flaxseed
5 dried figs
¼ cup agave
¼ cup honey
½ cup maple syrup
½ teaspoon Himalayan rock salt
Seeds of 1 vanilla pod

You'll need to make these the day before you want to eat them

Combine all the ingredients in a power blender, reserving ¼ cup goji berries to add in at the end. Turn out into a mixing bowl.

Add the ¼ cup soaked and drained goji berries into the mixing bowl and stir through.
Spread into rounds on the solid dehydrator sheets.
Dehydrate for 14–16 hours.

Take out of the dehydrator and top with fresh fruit and maca cream.

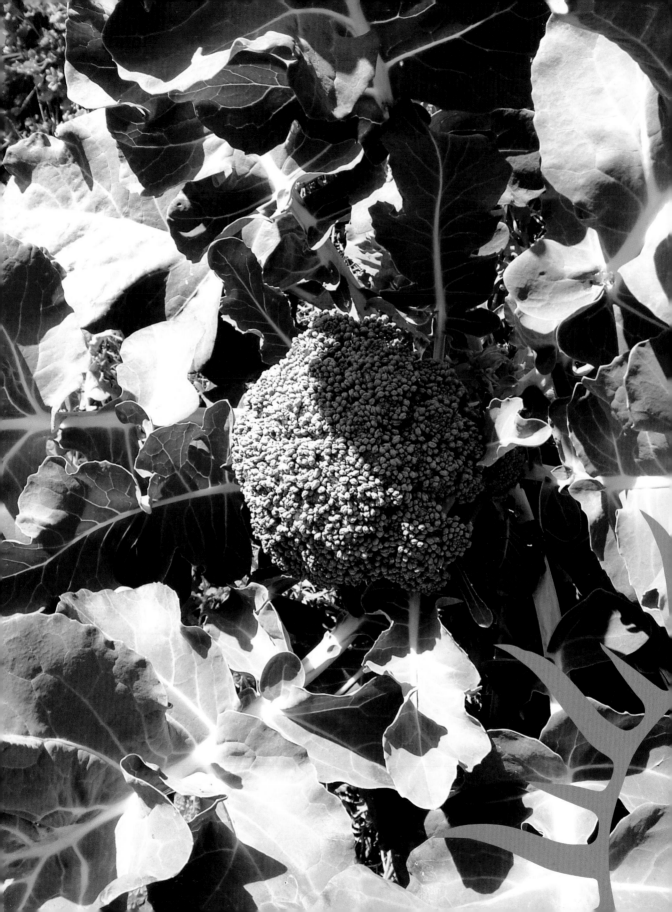

Soups

Warm Foods

Raw food doesn't have to mean cold food. Food that has not been heated above 116.6°F is still considered raw. This is because at 116.6°F and above the enzymes, minerals, vitamins, and phytonutrients in the food begin to denature. Eating raw soups is simply a continuation of the blender chef theme. All you do is throw your ingredients in a power blender and push the button.

There are a few ways to warm your soup.

1. *Friction*
The friction generated by your Vitamix or other power blender will eventually warm your soup.

2. *The kettle*
Parboil your kettle first and start with medium-hot water as your base.

3. *Stovetop*
Use the finger test – put your blended soup into a pot and warm it gently on the stovetop on low heat. As long as you can put your finger in the pot without being scorched you're still good to go.

Raw soups are comforting and warming, especially during winter. Liquidized foods digest easily, and will often take the stress off an overstrained digestive system. You could try giving your body a break from solid foods for a few days without having to starve yourself. Green vegetable juices, smoothies, and soups are delicious and nutritious alternatives to solid foods.

Another neat trick is to warm your bowls before serving the soup so that your soup stays warmer for longer while you are eating. You can do this by placing the bowls in the warming drawer of your oven or by pouring boiling water over the bowls.

Broccoli & Leek Soup

Serves 4

½ avocado
2 cups (500 mL) hot water
1 small head broccoli (approx 2 cups chopped)
4 medium-sized leek stalks
¼ cup (about 65 mL) olive oil
1 teaspoon Himalayan rock salt
1 tablespoon nutritional yeast
¼ cup pine nuts
¼ cup cashews
¼ cup sesame seeds

Blend all the ingredients except the sesame seeds until smooth.
Add the sesame seeds at the end and mix through.
Serve with a dollop of raw cream cheese
(see page 82) and a swirl of olive oil.
Garnish with a sprig of parsley.

*Broccoli contains
phytonutrients, which have
significant anti-cancer properties.*

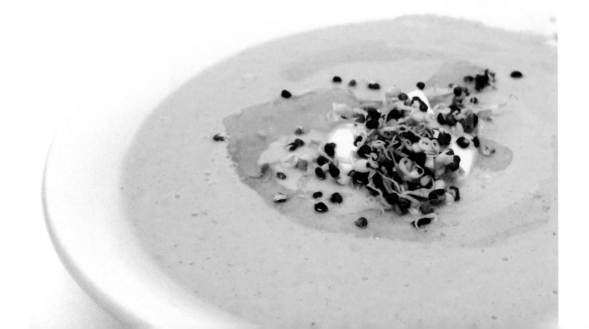

Red Bell Pepper & Tomato Soup

Serves 3–4

5 tomatoes
2 red bell peppers
¼ red onion
1 handful fresh basil leaves
1 handful cashews
2 tablespoons olive oil
Himalayan rock salt to taste
1 small handful goji berries
½ cup (125 mL) warm water
cayenne pepper to spice it up (optional)

Blend everything together. Add more water to achieve desired thickness.
Pour into soup bowls and enjoy.

Butternut-carrot-ginger Soup

Serves 3–4

1 cup (250 mL) carrot juice
2 cups butternut, roughly chopped
½ avocado
1 tablespoon olive oil
½ teaspoon Himalayan rock salt
½ cup (125 mL) apple juice
½ cup (125 mL) warm water
1 clove garlic
¼ cup cashews
½ inch (1 cm) piece ginger
1 teaspoon cumin
½ teaspoon cayenne pepper

Blend all the ingredients together in a power blender.

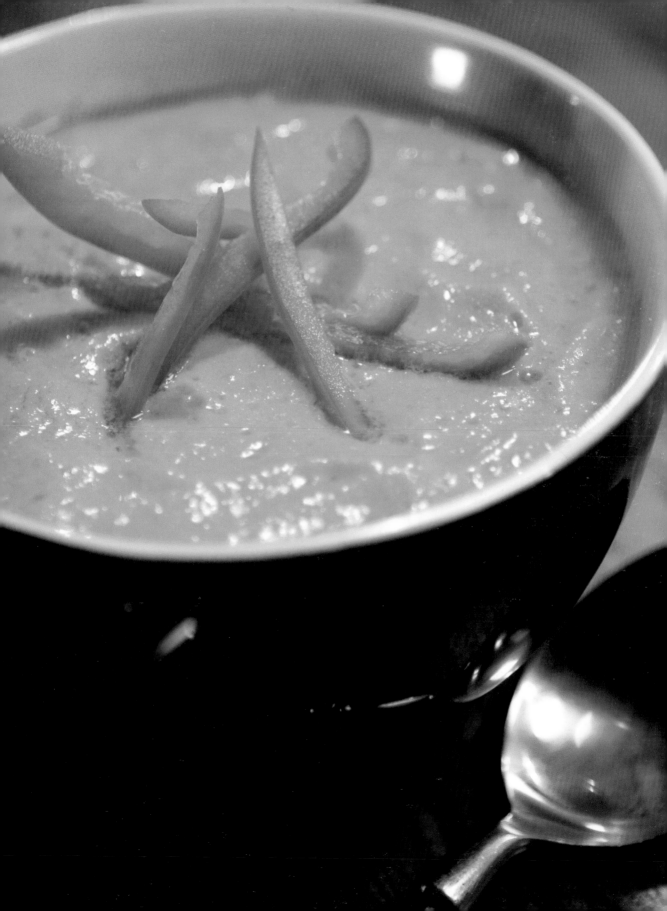

Mango-carrot-orange Soup

Serves 4–5

1½ cups (375 mL) carrot juice
1 cup (250 mL) orange juice
½ cup (125 mL) water
1 medium mango
2 tablespoons coconut cream
1 teaspoon cayenne pepper
½ teaspoon salt

Juice the carrots and oranges. Put the juice into your power blender and blend with the remaining ingredients. Blend until smooth and warm. Pour into bowls and serve.

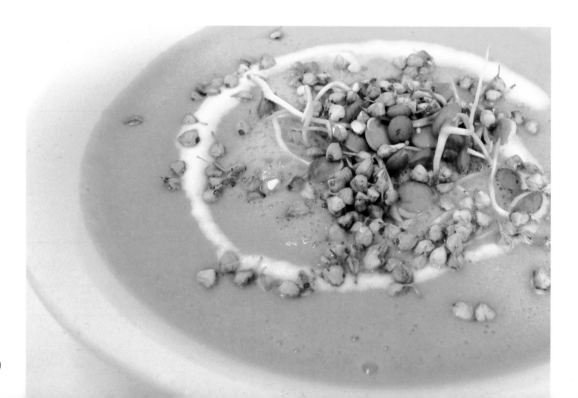

Miso Soup

Serves 3–4

4 cups (1 liter) warm water
2 tablespoons barley or brown rice miso
1 scallion, finely sliced
½ onion, finely diced
1 tablespoon olive oil
Selection of seaweeds
  2 strips kombu, sliced
  1 sheet nori, roughly torn
  5 strips dulse leaf
¼ teaspoon Himalayan rock salt
1 turnip

Miso is a salty-tasting fermented soybean paste originating in Japan. It can also be made from rice, barley, or wheat. When buying miso, look for an organic, unpasteurized brand.

Spiralize or grate the turnip to form noodles. Set it aside in a bowl and sprinkle with salt to soften. Blend the water, olive oil, salt, and miso together in a power blender. Add the onion, scallion, seaweeds, and turnip noodles and pulse briefly so that everything is mixed through but still floating in the broth.

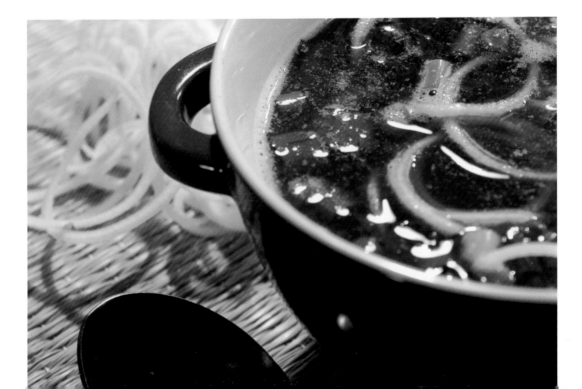

Wild Mushroom Soup

Serves 3–4

4 cups (1 liter) warm water
2 tablespoons barley or brown rice miso
1 teaspoon medicinal mushrooms
¼ onion
1 tablespoon olive oil
1 clove garlic
¼ cup macadamia nuts
2 tablespoons pine nuts
1 scallion, finely sliced
¼ cup parsley, roughly chopped
1 cup mixed wild mushrooms
   1 handful fresh king oyster mushrooms
   1 handful dried shiitakes or tree oyster mushrooms
   1 handful dried boletes mushrooms
½ teaspoon Himalayan rock salt
½ teaspoon black pepper

Medicinal mushrooms have been shown to boost the immune system, ward off viruses and bacteria, and combat allergies. Species that have demonstrated phenomenal healing potential include maitake, shiitake, reishi, coriolus, and agaricus blazei.

Blend the water, miso, medicinal mushrooms, onion, olive oil, salt, pine nuts, and macadamia nuts. Add the scallions and parsley and stir through. Add strips of wild mushrooms and stir again.

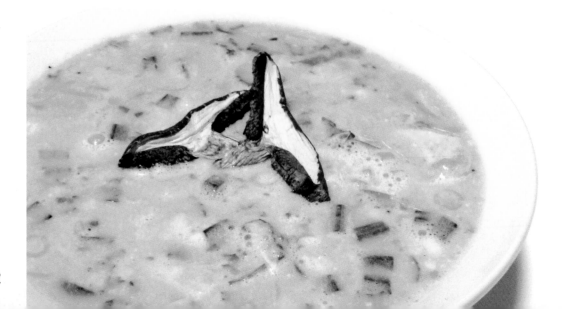

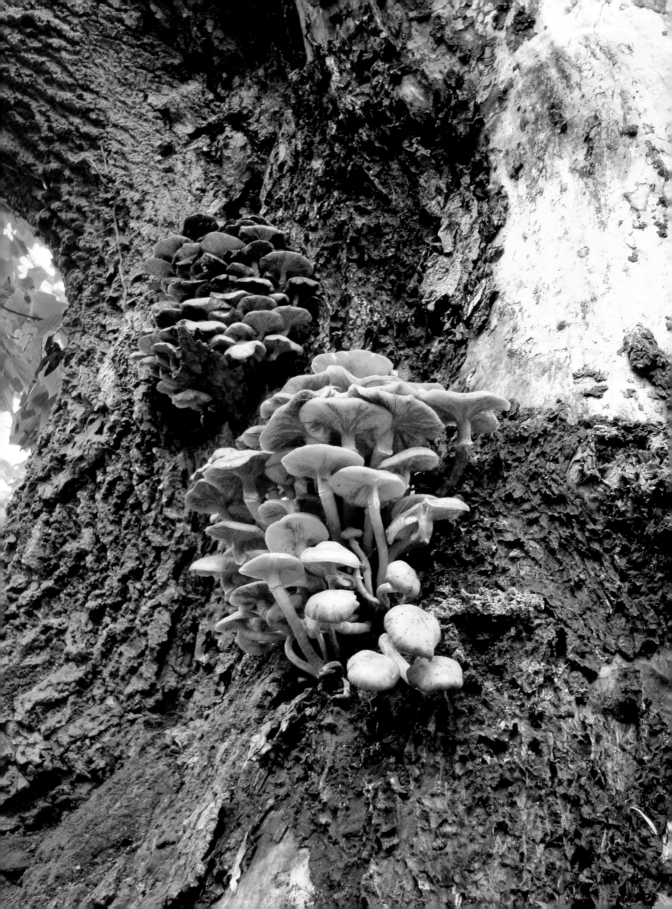

Cream of Celery Soup

Serves 4

2½ cups (625 mL) celery juice
1 cup (250 mL) water
2 scallions
1½ avocados
1 clove garlic
½ cup cilantro
¼ cup (about 65 mL) olive oil
¼ cup parsley
1 tablespoon lemon juice
1 teaspoon Himalayan rock salt

Blend all the ingredients together until a creamy consistency is reached. Avocados are a wonderful addition to raw soups as a way to thicken them up and give a creamier consistency.

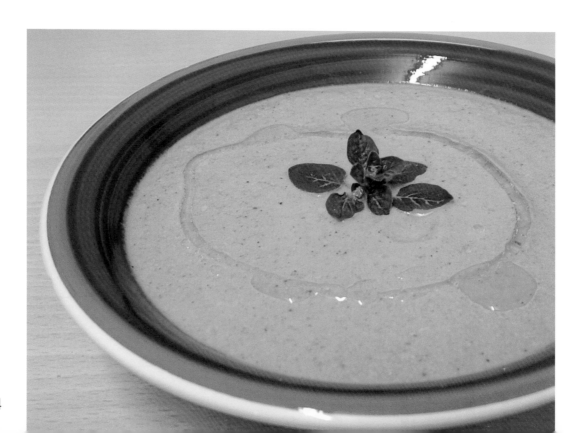

Liquid Salad Soup

Serves 4

At the beginning of this year I decided to do a one-week liquid feast. I created this soup by taking the ingredients that everyone else was using in their lunchtime salad and blending them instead. It was delicious and has remained a green soup favorite ever since.

2 sticks celery
½ cucumber
2 sprigs parsley
1 carrot
2 cups (500 mL) water
2 tablespoons Bragg Liquid Aminos
2 teaspoons miso
1 handful arugula
2½ oz (75 g) sunflower sprouts (or other salad greens)
3 spinach leaves
1 nori sheet
2 tablespoons olive oil
½ red onion
1 small clove garlic
1 avocado
1 teaspoon salt
1 handful cashews

Juice the celery, cucumber, parsley, and carrots. Place the juice in a blender with the rest of the ingredients and blend until smooth. Serve warm or cold, topped with sprouts and a swirl of olive oil.

If you aren't used to eating green leaves, blending them is another great way to add them to your diet without having to juice them.

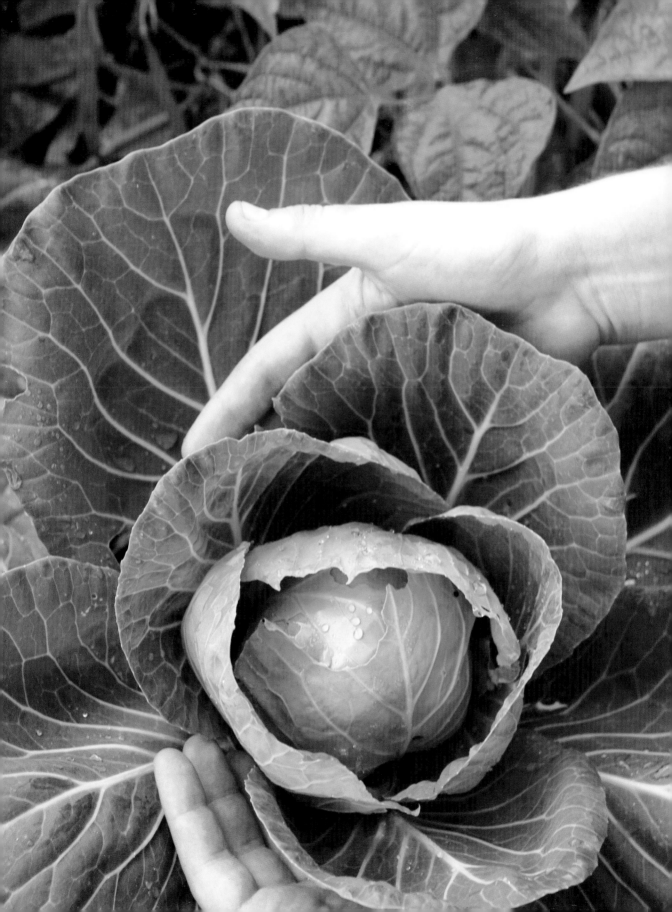

Salads

Salad Construction

Learning to love a good salad is vital to succeeding on a high-percentage raw food diet. We have a salad every day, usually at lunchtime. Peter's lunchtime salad bowl is the size most people would serve as a table salad for three or four people. Nutritionally, green leaves are the correct foods for our bodies, so the more we get in the better.

One of the biggest problems people have with salads is that they think of a salad as a combination of iceberg lettuce, tomato and cucumber. That is not a salad – at least, not in my book. I'm talking about a real salad – one that is overflowing with organic, mineral-rich and flavorful leaves, sprouts, nuts, seeds, fruits, and vegetables. When Peter and I first met he never used to eat my salads. He would push the leaves to the edge of his plate and refer to them as "tasteless fiber and water." It was only when we switched to organic produce that the greens started to take center stage on his plate and the meat and cooked foods slowly edged their way off entirely.

Something to bear in mind is that if you've been only eating cooked foods, the fiber in salads can be difficult to digest at first. The digestive system becomes weakened by lack of exercise and years of cooked food abuse, so chewing your salads properly is essential.

There are a few tricks to a making a great raw salad. Firstly, use organic leaves – they always taste better. The darker and greener the leaves are, the more chlorophyll they contain and therefore the more alkalizing they are for your body. Sprouts are the only food that is still growing when you eat it. The more homegrown foods and sprouts you eat, the better you will feel. Once you've got a nice bed of high-quality green leaves, add some fresh tomatoes and cucumber. To this gorgeous salad base, add foods that are rich in good fats and will give substance to your salad such as avocados, olives, nuts, and seeds. Add a variety of flavorful herbs such as parsley, cilantro, or basil. Finally, create variations by adding something different such as sauces, pestos, and dressings or simply drizzle your salad with olive oil and lemon juice. Top it all off with a sprinkling of Himalayan rock salt or cracked black pepper.

Here's what eating salads daily has to offer you nutritionally:

The rich green salad leaves are high in alkalizing chlorophyll, magnesium, and free-form amino acids or proteins. They are also high in silica, which is good for the hair, skin, and nails. They have an abundance of vitamins and minerals, including trace minerals. They are a source of high-quality water and essential fiber. Fiber gets the digestive system moving again and, contrary to popular belief, does not only come in brown boxes and taste like cardboard.

Sprouts are a living food and help facilitate detoxification, alkalization, and weight loss. Broccoli contains iron and is helpful for relieving high blood pressure and constipation. Olives contain good levels of protein, are one of the top mucus-dissolving foods, and are a great source of essential fatty acids. Avocados are delicious and are also an excellent source of good fats. Himalayan rock salt and sea salt contain vital trace minerals.

Salads are as much a feast for the stomach as for the eyes. Falling in love with fresh salads is one of the most delightful culinary affairs you can have, not just with the raw ingredients themselves but with their colors, contrasts, and textures too.

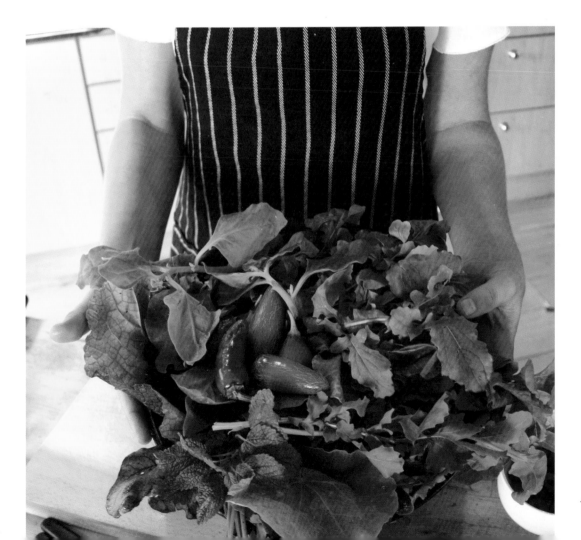

Green Staples:

Everyday Green Salad

A selection of:
lettuce greens, arugula, spinach
sprouts
cucumber
tomato
avocado

Assemble a generous amount of all these ingredients in a salad bowl. Use some of the following additions to make the salad even more interesting:

olives
mixed seeds (see page 144)
broccoli chips (see page 146)
buckwheaties (see page 147)

Top with dressing of choice (see page 135).

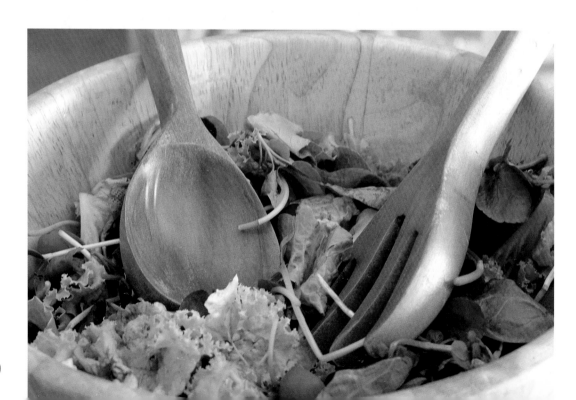

Kale & Baby Spinach Salad

Serves 3–4

This is a definite favorite among raw foodies.

1½ cup kale, destalked, and cut into strips
2 cups baby spinach
1 tablespoon lemon juice
1 tablespoon apple cider vinegar
2 medium avocados
½ teaspoon Himalayan rock salt
1 cup alfalfa sprouts
½ grapefruit, sliced

Take the kale strips and baby spinach and massage the avocado and all the other ingredients, excluding the alfalfa and the grapefruit, into the leaves. Use your hands to mix everything together thoroughly and love your food as you do so. Your hands will love you for it, too. Garnish with alfalfa sprouts and sliced grapefruit.

The avocado and vinegar combination is very moisturizing to the hands because of the good oils in the avocado and the acidity in the vinegar.

Super Simple Sprout Salad

Serves 2

This is one of my favorite supper snacks. It's quick, it's easy, it's nutritious, and it fills the gap in the evening when I don't want to eat a big meal but also don't want to skip dinner altogether.

2 cups of your favorite mixed sprouts
½ avocado, diced
1 tomato, diced
1 tablespoon tamari sauce
1 pinch Himalayan rock salt

Mix all the ingredients together in a bowl and enjoy this super simple living salad!

Make sure that you have a variety of sprouts on the go.

Our Favorites

Here is a selection of some of our favorite raw salads with contributions made by some close friends.

Beryn's Sunflower Sprout Salad

Serves 4

This salad came about one day when I got home from a holiday and there were no fresh greens in the house. I was stumped for a moment and then realized I had carrots, cabbages, and some sunflower greens growing outside. It took less than ten minutes to assemble this salad and I went through a phase of making it every single day for about two weeks after that. The carrots, sunflower greens, and gooseberries make a really colorful feast for the eyes and a perfect table salad for when you have people over.

1 cup sunflower greens
1 cup mixed sprouts
½ baby cabbage, grated
2 carrots, grated
1 handful walnuts
sprinkling of chopped dried figs
1½–2 avocados, diced
½ cup baby tomatoes
1 handful gooseberries
parsley to garnish

Grate the carrots and cabbage first.
Combine the carrot, cabbage, sprouts,
dried fruit, baby tomatoes, and walnuts.
Top with diced avocado and gooseberries.
Garnish with finely chopped parsley.

Optional: Drizzle with a simple salad dressing
of olive oil, lemon juice, and honey.

Sunflower greens are one of the most nutritionally dense greens, and can be easily grown at home. Sunflower greens are almost 25 percent protein and are a rich source of lecithin, which helps digest fats.

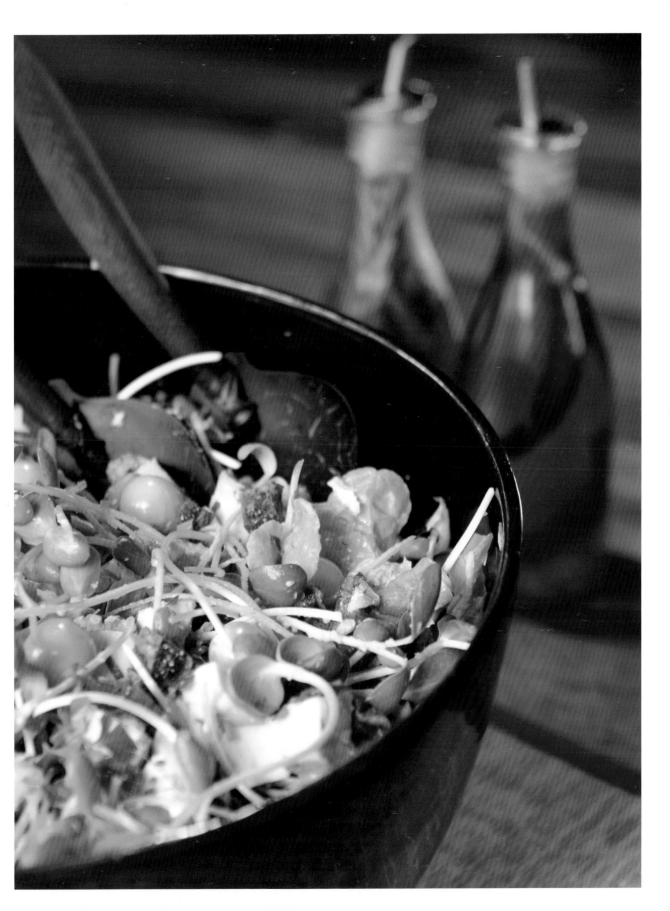

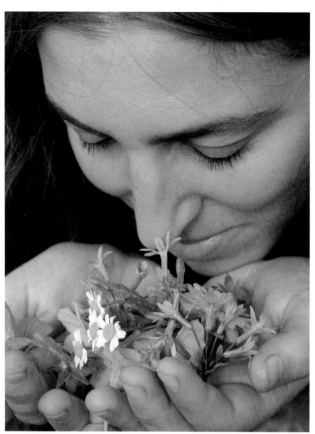
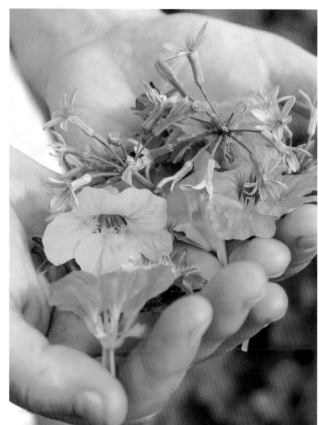
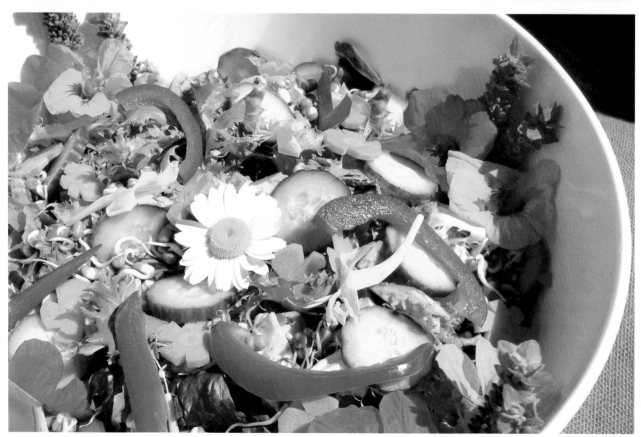

Wild Lexi's Flower Power Salad

Lexi is a true artist – she can take an everyday green salad and bring it to life by spending ten minutes wandering around the garden picking whatever edible flowers are available. You would be amazed at how many edible flowers there are and what a difference they make to an otherwise ordinary salad.

Take your Everyday Green Salad ingredients (see page 110)
Add sliced red bell peppers and a mix of the following flowers:

Nasturtium flowers
Daisy petals
Marigold petals
Borage flowers
Garlic chive flowers
Fennel flowers
Geranium flowers
Arugula flowers
Clover flowers
Mint flowers
Cilantro flowers
Basil flowers
Thyme flowers
Zucchini flowers
Butternut squash flowers

Go hunting for wild and edible flowers

All edible plants and herbs have edible flowers, though some may taste a bit strong and medicinal. In springtime, flowers should form a massive part of our natural diet, as they are truly abundant and springing up all around us.

Spending ten minutes walking around your garden barefoot and picking flowers could potentially be more nourishing, relaxing, and grounding for your being than the eating of the food itself.

Barbara's Subtle Salad

Barbara is another one our favorite friends and a fellow raw food enthusiast. She loves to spend time in the kitchen experimenting with different dishes and flavors. One evening at her place she served up this divine salad. It was light and the flavors were subtle and scrumptious, so we named it Barbara's Subtle Salad.

Dark greens like New Zealand spinach, swiss chard, arugula, and other lettuce varieties, finely shredded
walnuts or pecans
raisins
1 seasonal fruit
sprouts
sundried tomatoes, finely sliced

The key to this salad is to slice the ingredients finely. Combine everything in a big salad bowl and toss with a little bit of lemon juice.

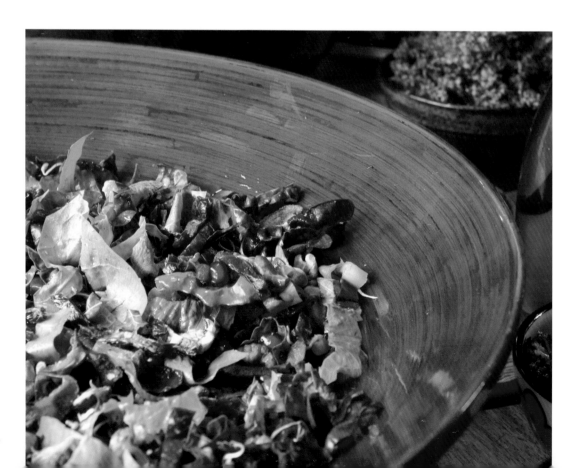

Mom's Three Bean Salad

Serves 2–3

Peter's mom has always made a traditional three-bean salad using tinned beans and a sugary salad dressing. One day when we were visiting, we decided to convert this family favorite into a raw, healthy version. We simply took the old recipe, substituted the tinned ingredients with fresh sprouted beans and replaced the sugar and white vinegar in the dressing for healthy alternatives.

1 cup mixed pea sprouts
½ cup mung beans
1 cup string beans, chopped
½ cup adzuki beans

Dressing:
¼ cup apple cider vinegar
¼ cup olive oil
⅛ cup honey
2 tablespoons fresh chopped parsley
2 tablespoons fresh chopped basil
½ teaspoon mustard powder
½ teaspoon Himalayan rock salt
¼ teaspoon black pepper
1 clove garlic, crushed

This salad tastes better if you allow it to stand in the fridge & infuse with the dressing for 3 hours.

Put the mix of beans and sprouts into a salad bowl. Make the dressing by putting all the remaining ingredients in a glass jar and shaking them up. Pour the dressing over the salad and let stand in the refrigerator for 3 hours to infuse.

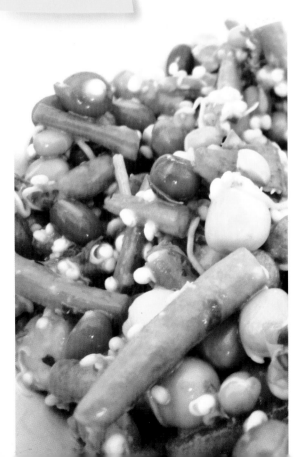

117

Coleslaws

Coleslaws are a great way to get root veggies and cabbages into your salads and put a variety of flavors and colors on the table. They're especially nourishing for winter.

Cabbage Mayo Coleslaw

Serves 2–3

2 cups green cabbage, grated
2 cups red cabbage, grated
½ white onion, chopped
sprinkling Himalayan rock salt
¼ cup (about 65 mL) apple cider vinegar
Mock Mayo (see page 131)

Combine the cabbages and onion in a salad bowl. Make up a batch of mayo (see page 131), pour over the salad, and mix through.

Thai Coleslaw

Serves 3–4

2 cups red cabbage, grated
2 cups green cabbage, grated
2 cups thinly grated zucchini (approx 3 zucchini)
1½ cups grated carrots (approx 2–3 carrots)
½ onion chopped
2 scallions, finely sliced
1 cup loosely packed cilantro, then chopped
⅓ cup cashew nuts
1 tablespoon black sesame seeds
Thai Sauce (see page 132)

Grate the cabbages, carrots, and zucchini together, chop the onions and combine in a salad bowl with the scallion, cilantro, and cashews. Make a batch of the Thai Sauce from the sauces section (see page 132), pour over the salad, and mix well. Sprinkle the black sesame seeds on top with a few extra cashew nuts.

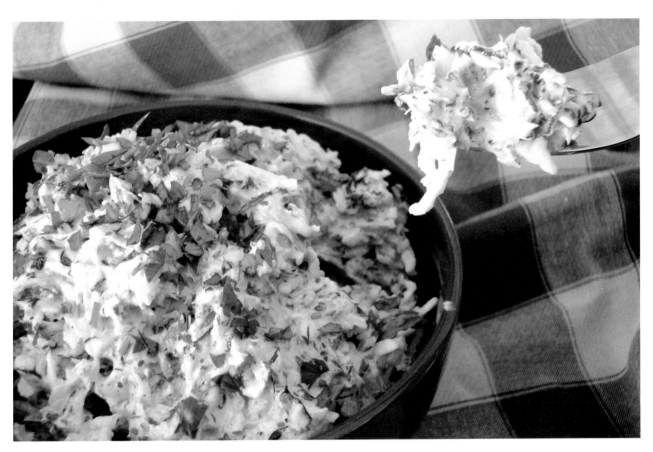

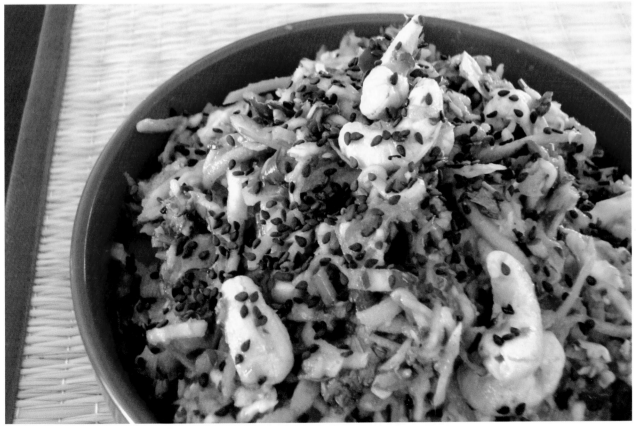

Beet and Carrot Salad

Serves 3–4

4 beets, peeled
4 carrots, peeled
1 tablespoon Braggs liquid aminos or tamari sauce
dash of olive oil
1 large handful small black currants or raisins
1 large handful pine nuts
Himalayan rock salt to taste
1 handful goji berries, soaked (optional)

Grate the beets and carrots into a salad bowl.
Add the other ingredients and toss.

Carrots really are good f
the eyes. They also help
reduce inflammation of t
mucus membranes in th
intestines and respirato
tract. Beet is an excellen
blood builder.

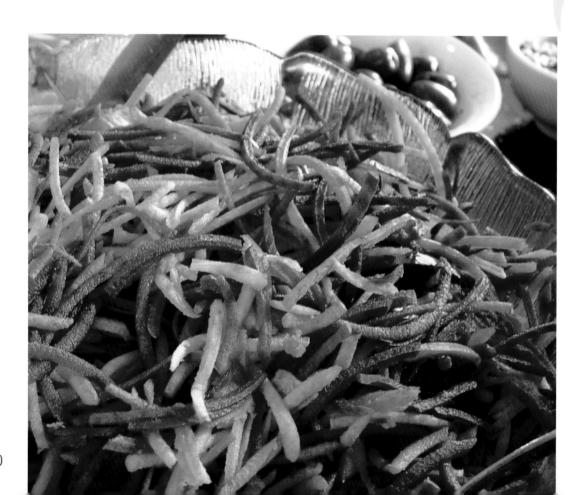

Sprouted Salads

Sprouted foods are always better for your health than nonsprouted foods. These two recipes are raw versions of their cooked counterparts, which are definitely better for you and taste better, too.

Sprouted Quinoa Salad

Serves 4

3 cups sprouted quinoa (see page 24)
1 cup finely chopped parsley
2 tablespoons fresh chopped basil
1 tablespoon garlic chives
⅛ cup (65 mL) olive oil
1 cup baby tomatoes
1 tablespoon tamari sauce
½ teaspoon Himalayan rock salt
Juice of ½ lemon

Place all the ingredients in a large salad bowl and toss.

Start soaking & sprouting your quinoa 2 days earlier

Quinoa (pronounced Keen-wah) is a recently rediscovered ancient seed/grain native to South America. Not only is quinoa high in protein, but the protein it supplies is complete protein, meaning that it includes all nine essential amino acids.

Sprouted Chickpea Salad

Serves 6

5 cups sprouted chickpeas (see page 24)
1 tablespoon tamari
4 tablespoons olive oil
½ cup fresh cilantro, finely chopped
¾ cup sundried tomatoes, thinly sliced
1 tablespoon lemon juice
2 cloves garlic, finely chopped
Himalayan rock salt to taste
2 avocados, cubed

Combine all ingredients except the avocado in a large salad bowl. Top with cubed pieces of avocado and serve with a green salad.

Chickpeas take 2–3 days to sprout.

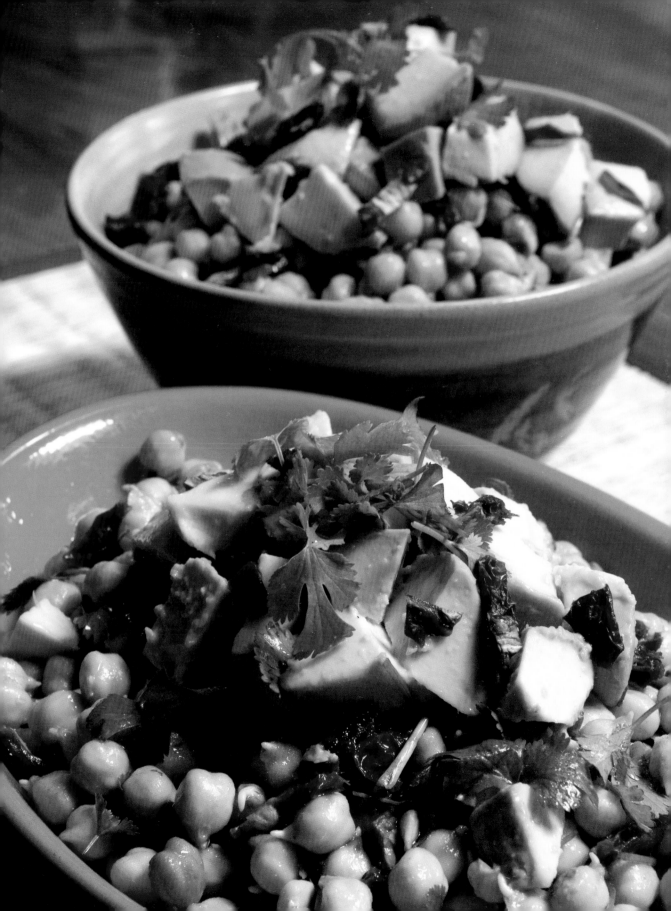

Seaweed Salad

Sea vegetables can be described as the last bastion of original food. They haven't been tampered with or altered by cross-breeding or genetic modification. They are a true heirloom food source that is packed with minerals and trace minerals. The sea contains all 92 minerals needed for real nutrition and the plants that grow in the sea have access to all of them.

This salad is more of a side or accompaniment to a main course salad but adding it will increase the nutrient density of your meal by miles.

3½ oz (100 g) bag of wakame (presoaked for at least 30 minutes to soften)
2 tablespoons tamari sauce
2 tablespoons honey
1 tablespoon lemon juice
1 teaspoon olive oil
1 small clove garlic, finely chopped
1 inch (about 2 cm) piece ginger, finely chopped

Drain the wakame and chop into rough, bite-sized pieces.
Place in a bowl and mix through with all the other ingredients.
It can be eaten straight away but the flavors will infuse best if you allow it to marinate for about 30 minutes.

Soak the Wakame for 30 minutes

Seaweed offers the broadest range of minerals of any food, containing virtually all the minerals found in the ocean – and the same minerals that are found in human blood.

Creamed Asparagus

Serves 3–4

14 oz (about 400 g) asparagus, chopped
⅓ cup (about 85 mL) apple cider vinegar
¼ cup tahini
2 cloves garlic
1 tablespoon lemon juice
¼ cup olive oil
¼ teaspoon salt

Place all the dressing ingredients in a bowl and stir thoroughly with a fork. Add the chopped asparagus to the dressing and stir through till well coated. Serve with a green salad.

"Tuna" Mayo

Serves 3–4

3 cups sunflower seeds, soaked and rinsed
4 stalks celery, diced
½ bunch scallions, diced
¼ cup fresh parsley, finely chopped
sprinkling of kelp
Mock Mayo (see page 131)

Make up a batch of mayonnaise

Grind the sunflower seeds in a food processor.
Combine with the other base ingredients above.
Make up a batch of mayo (see page 131), pour over the base salad ingredients, and mix well.

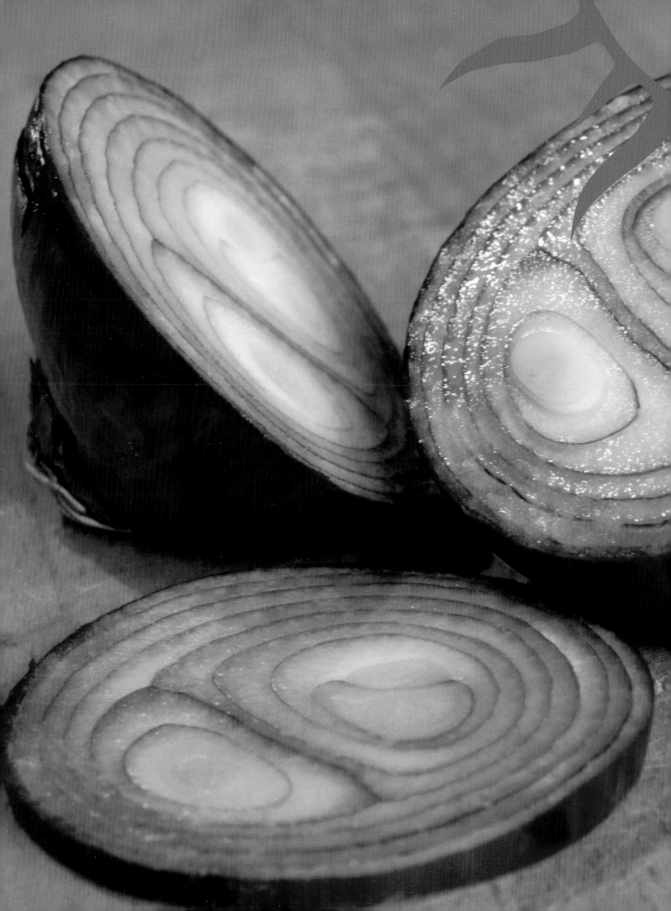

Sauces & Dressings

Tomato Sauce

Olive Tapenade

Basil Pesto

Cilantro Pesto

Sprouted Chickpea Hummus

Dairy-free Garlic Butter

Garlic White Sauce

Tahina

Mock Mayo

Thai Sauce

Almond Gravy

Indian Korma Sauce

Simple Salad Dressing

Infused Salad Dressings

Bell Pepper, Almond, and Ginger Dressing

This section on sauces and dressings may be one of the most valuable chapters to get your head around.

A simple sauce or dressing can take almost no time at all to prepare and can change the taste, texture, and look of a salad or simple meal into something a whole lot more gourmet. Many of these recipes can be made on a day when you have some spare time and stored in glass jars and refrigerated or even frozen so that when you need them or feel like something slightly different they are ready and waiting for you.

The equipment you will need to make the recipes in this section will be a food processor or a power blender. Whenever I mention using a power blender it is because I want the sauce to come out creamy and smooth. You may need to use the tamper to achieve this. In all instances you can use a food processor instead, but the texture will vary a little and become more chunky. No doubt it will still be delicious.

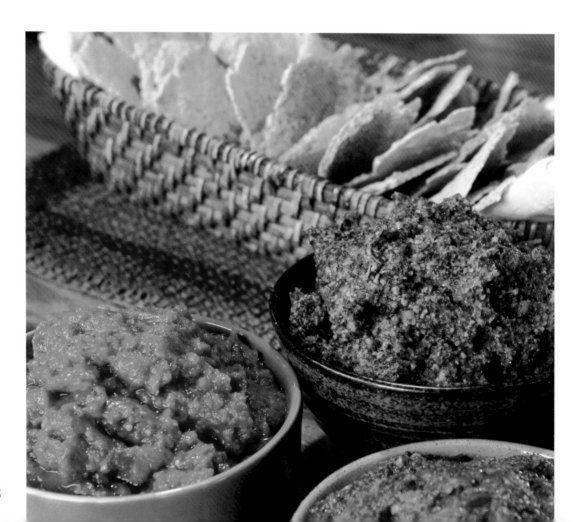

Sauces

Tomato Sauce

1 cup fresh tomatoes
½ cup sundried tomatoes
1 clove garlic
1 tablespoon olive oil
4 pitted dates or 1 teaspoon honey
Himalayan rock salt to taste

Halve the fresh tomatoes, put them in your power blender with the remaining ingredients, and blend until smooth.

Olive Tapenade

1 cup pitted olives
1 small mild chili pepper
½ clove garlic
Handful sundried tomatoes (optional)

Combine all the ingredients in a power blender or food processor.

Basil Pesto

Pesto freezes well, so make a big batch and store.

3 cups fresh basil
1 clove garlic
⅓ cup macadamia nuts
⅓ cup pumpkin seeds
⅛ cup lemon juice
½ teaspoon salt
⅓ cup (about 85 mL) olive oil

In a food processor blend all the ingredients until well chopped and combined.

Cilantro Pesto

2 cups fresh cilantro
1 cup arugula
2 cloves garlic
⅓ cup brazil nuts
⅓ cup sunflower seeds
⅓ cup pumpkin seeds
⅔ cup (165 mL) olive oil
4 tablespoons lemon juice
½ teaspoon kelp powder
Himalayan rock salt to taste

Place all the ingredients in a food processor or power blender and blend until everything is well combined.

Sprouted Chickpea Hummus

2 cups sprouted chickpeas
½ cup tahini
½ cup (125 mL) water
2 cloves garlic
2 tablespoons lemon juice
Himalyan rock salt to taste

Blend all the ingredients in a power blender or food processor until smooth.

Dairy-free Garlic Butter

olive oil
coconut oil
turmeric
garlic
Himalayan rock salt

In a small bowl mix equal quantities of olive oil and melted coconut oil. Add a pinch of turmeric powder for color, crushed garlic, and salt to taste. Refrigerate until set.

Garlic White Sauce

¾ cup macadamia nuts
4 cloves garlic
Juice of 1 lemon
1½ teaspoons salt
3 tablespoons olive oil
1 cup (250 mL) water

Blend all the ingredients in a power blender.

Tahina

1 cup tahini
¾ cup (about 190 mL) water
¼ cup (about 65 mL) lemon juice
½ clove garlic
2 teaspoons Himalayan rock salt
⅛ red onion

Blend everything together in a food processor or blender. Add more water if necessary to get the right creamy consistency.

Tahini is sesame seed butter; sesame seeds are very high in calcium.

Mock Mayo

½ cup cashew nuts
½ cup macadamia nuts
½ cup (125 mL) water
½ tablespoon apple cider vinegar
3 tablespoons olive oil
3 pitted dates
1 tablespoon tamari
1 tablespoon lemon juice
1 clove garlic
¼ teaspoon Himalayan rock salt

Place all the ingredients in a power blender and blend well.
To make sour cream remove the apple cider vinegar, dates, garlic, and tamari sauce.

Thai Sauce

1 red bell pepper
1 cup (250 mL) olive oil
1 teaspoon chili flakes or cayenne pepper (more if you like it very hot)
2 tablespoons lemon juice
2 tablespoons apple cider vinegar
3 tablespoons tamari
1½ tablespoons honey
3 cloves garlic
1 inch (about 2 cm) piece ginger, peeled
1 teaspoon curry powder
1 tablespoon cilantro
½ teaspoon Himalayan rock salt

Blend all the ingredients together in a power blender.

Almond Gravy

1 cup almonds
⅓ cup tamari
1 tablespoon tahini
1 cup (250 mL) water

Blend all the ingredients together in a power blender.

Indian Korma Sauce

8 tomatoes
1 red onion
1 inch (about 2 cm) piece ginger
3 cloves garlic
½ teaspoon turmeric
2 teaspoons curry powder
½ teaspoon cayenne pepper
½ teaspoon ground cinnamon
1 teaspoon Himalayan rock salt
¼ cup (about 65 mL) olive oil
½ cup dried peaches
¼ cup sundried tomatoes, sliced
¼ cup dried figs (or pitted dates)
½ cup (125 mL) coconut milk
½ cup cashew nuts
½ cup macadamia nuts

Garnish with:
cilantro, yellow and red bell pepper

Blend all the ingredients together in a power blender.
To make a meal of this sauce, serve it with turnip rice (see page 154) and finely sliced spinach.

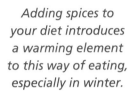

Adding spices to your diet introduces a warming element to this way of eating, especially in winter.

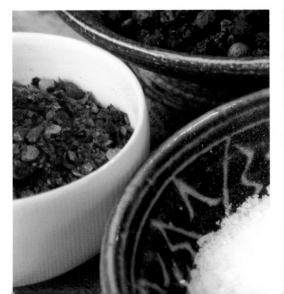

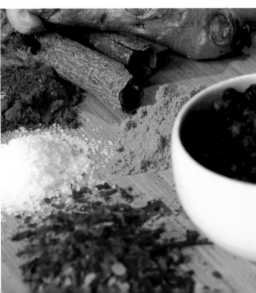

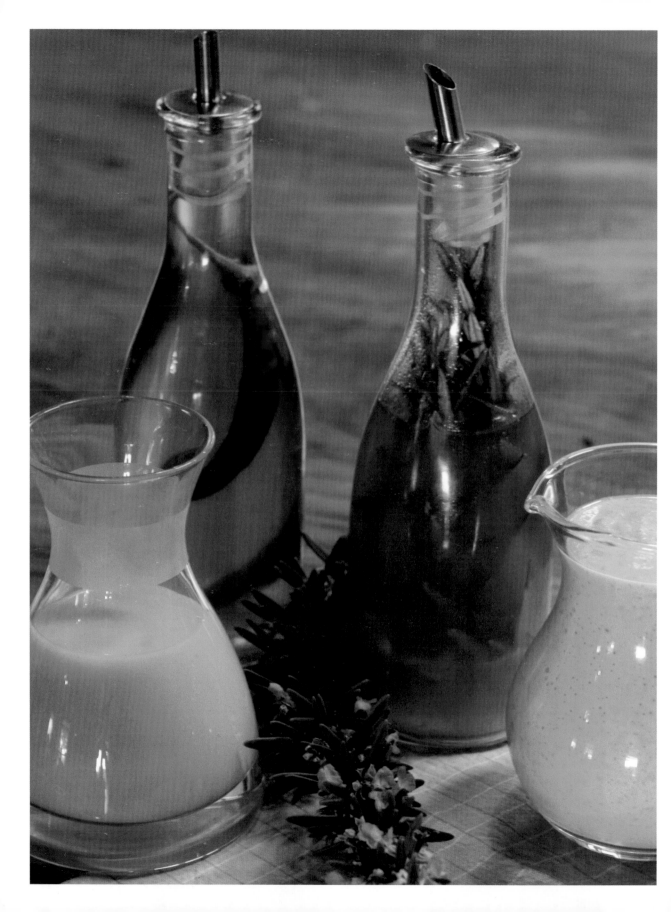

Dressings

To make a good basic salad dressing you will need the following:
something fatty: e.g., olive oil, nuts, or avocados
something tart: e.g., apple cider vinegar or lemon juice
something sweet: e.g., honey, agave, or sweet fruits
something salty: e.g., Himalayan rock salt or tamari sauce

Simple Salad Dressing

½ cup (125 mL) olive oil
Juice of 1 lemon
3 tablespoons honey
3 tablespoons apple cider vinegar
Himalayan rock salt
1 tablespoon tamari sauce (optional)

Put all the ingredients into a glass jar and shake vigorously.

Infused Salad Dressings

Take the dressing above and add any of the following ingredients and allow to infuse.

whole chilis or ginger slices
garlic cloves or rosemary sprigs

Bell Pepper, Almond & Ginger Dressing

1 red bell pepper
1 inch (about 2 cm) piece ginger
Juice of 1 orange
¼ cup almonds
3 tablespoons olive oil
1 tablespoon lemon juice
1 teaspoon apple cider vinegar
½ teaspoon Himalayan rock salt

Blend all the ingredients together in a power blender.

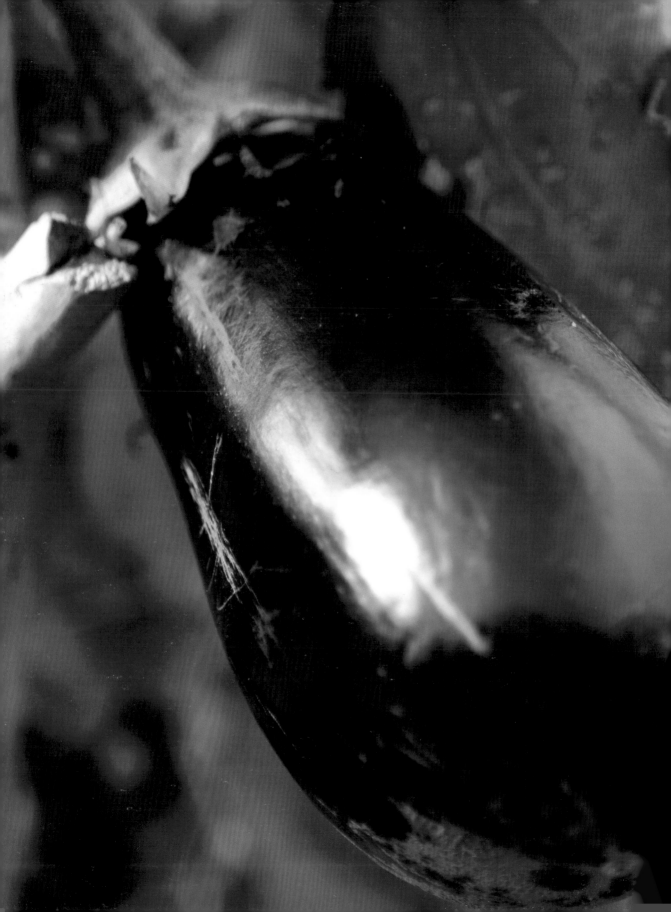

Sides & Snacks

Guacamole

Creamed Spinach

Salsa

Mango Atchar

"Egg" Mayo

Marinated Onions

Hemp & Pumpkin Seed Pâté

Marinated Mixed Bell Peppers & Tomatoes

Cucumber, Avocado & Dulse/Olive Bites

Spiced Mixed Seeds

Sweet Chili Cashews

Pesto-stuffed Mushrooms

Broccoli Chips

Eggplant Jerky

Buckwheaties

Superfood Trail Mix

Nutty Dates

Dried Fruit

Dripping Dried Figs

Cookies

This chapter is made up of sides, savory snacks, and sweet snacks. Each of the side dishes are best eaten in conjunction with a nice big green salad. My best way to eat these dishes is to make up two or three different types of sides and enjoy them meze-style with one or two different types of salad. I usually prepare the savory snacks either as canapés or to use as additions to simple salads. The sweet snacks are a variety of good healthy options to satisfy that sweet tooth craving.

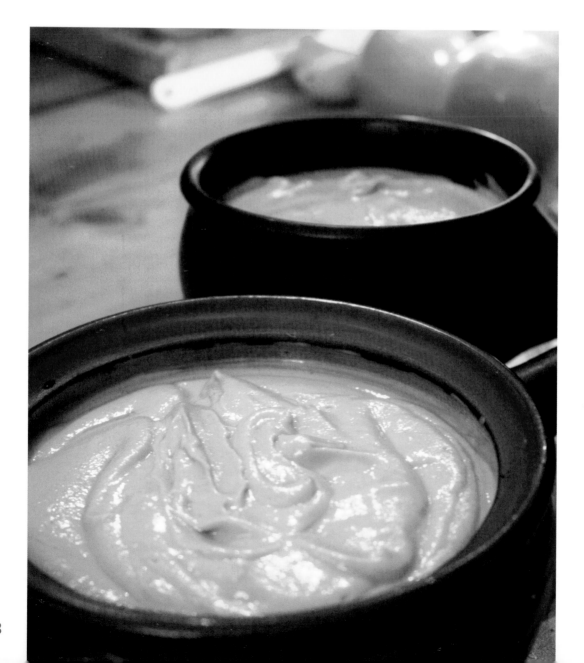

Sides

Guacamole

Mmmm, my favorite dish of all time (after chocolate mousse).

2 large avocados
⅛ cup olive oil
1 scallion
1 handful cilantro
1 lemon, juiced
Himalayan rock salt to taste

Put all ingredients into your power blender or food processor and blend until smooth and creamy.

Creamed Spinach

Take a bunch of spinach, roughly chopped. Place in a bowl and sprinkle with salt. The salt will wilt the spinach. Allow to stand for a few minutes then squeeze any excess liquid off the spinach. Take your instant cashew nut cheese or cream cheese (see page 90) and mix through with the wilted spinach to give you a creamy texture.

Salsa

5–6 fresh tomatoes
½ cup cilantro
½ fresh chili
2 tablespoons lemon juice
½ red onion
Himalayan rock salt to taste

Add all ingredients to your food processor and use the pulse on/off button to process the ingredients until well combined and chunky, but not completely smooth.

Mango Atchar

1 large mango, cut into small chunks
½ cup dried peaches
¼ cup goji berries
Juice of 1 lemon
Juice of 1 orange
4 medium tomatoes
1 medium red onion
½ cup fresh cilantro
1 clove garlic
1 teaspoon cayenne pepper
1 teaspoon curry masala
½ teaspoon salt
1 tablespoon honey
Scallions to garnish

Soak the goji berries and dried peaches in the lemon and orange juice.
Place all the ingredients except the mango chunks in the food processor and process until roughly chopped. Add the mango and pulse it through. Garnish with scallion slices and serve.

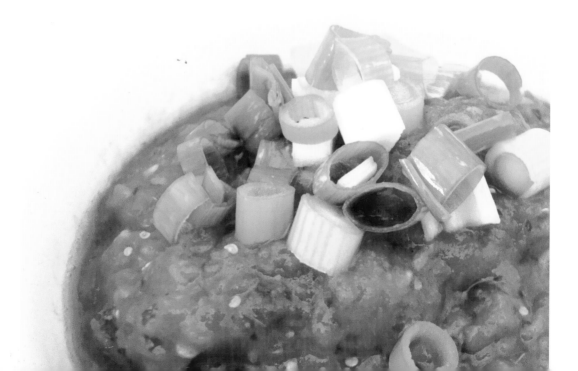

"Egg" Mayo

I started making this recipe when I discovered black Indian salt; it has a strong sulfur scent and makes this dish smell and taste like egg mayonnaise.

½ cup (125 mL) water
½ cup (125 mL) lemon juice
1½ teaspoons turmeric
1 clove garlic
1½ cups macadamia or cashew nuts
1 teaspoon black Indian salt
½ cup chopped scallion
½ cup chopped celery
½ cup chopped red bell pepper

In a high-speed blender combine the first six ingredients. Put the mixture in a bowl and add the scallion, celery, and red bell pepper. Mix well and serve.

Marinated Onions

3 red onions
3 tablespoons olive oil
2 tablespoons tamari
1 tablespoon apple cider vinegar

Cut the onions into thinly sliced rings or using a spiralizer with no extra fittings, make onion noodles. Place the onions in a bowl and coat with the olive oil, tamari, and vinegar. Place them in the dehydrator on a solid sheet for at least 5–6 hours. The longer you leave them the crispier they get.

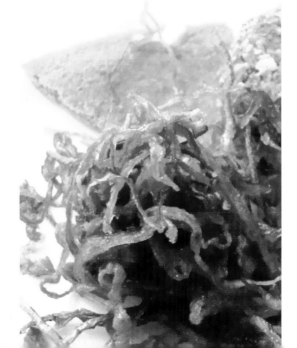

Hemp & Pumpkin Seed Pâté

1 cup pumpkin seeds, soaked
¼ cup sundried tomatoes, soaked
⅛ cup almonds or pine nuts
1 clove garlic
2 tablespoons olive oil
2 tablespoons hemp protein powder
1 tablespoon lemon juice
1 teaspoon Himalayan rock salt
1 teaspoon dried mixed herbs

Hemp seeds and pumpkin seeds are two of the highest protein-content seeds.

Combine all the ingredients together in your food processor.
Add water if the pâté is too thick.

Marinated Mixed Bell Peppers & Tomatoes

A great way to use excess produce is to dehydrate, marinate, and store it for later.

4–5 mixed bell peppers, sliced
10 fresh tomatoes, cut into wedges
garlic cloves, sliced
olive oil
apple cider vinegar
Himalayan rock salt

Dehydrate the bell peppers and garlic for 4–5 hours. The tomatoes can go for up to 24 hours or until almost completely dry. Put all the dehydrated items in a glass jar and drizzle with olive oil, apple cider, vinegar, and salt.

Dehydrate your excess produce & use as great salad extras.

Savory Snacks

Cucumber, Avocado & Dulse/Olive Bites

cucumber, sliced into rounds or mandolined into thin strips
avocado, diced
dulse strips or pitted olives
chives

Place the cucumber rounds on a plate and top with a square of avocado and a slither of dulse or a pitted olive.

Alternative preparation:
Take a mandolined cucumber strip, place a piece of avocado at the base of the strip, and cover with a strip of dulse or a pitted olive. Slowly roll the cucumber strip up and hold it together by tying it closed with a chive.

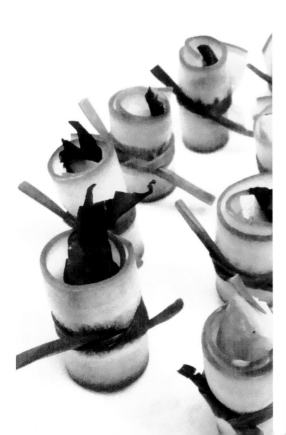
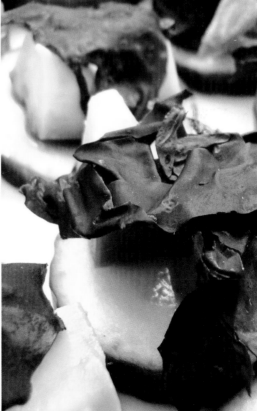

Spiced Mixed Seeds

2 cups sunflower seeds, soaked and rinsed
1 cup pumpkin seeds
¼ cup tamari sauce
1 tablespoon maple syrup or honey
1 tablespoon ground cumin
1 teaspoon garlic powder
2 tablespoons apple cider vinegar
½ teaspoon cayenne pepper
1 teaspoon whole cilantro seeds, crushed in a coffee grinder
1 teaspoon curry powder

Mix all the ingredients together in a bowl.
Dehydrate for 18–24 hours or until dry and crunchy.
Stores well in glass jars.

Sweet Chili Cashews

2 cups cashews
2 tablespoons honey
½ teaspoon salt
1 teaspoon cayenne pepper
1 teaspoon curry powder

Make a blend of honey, salt, and spices. Add a little water if required. Roll the cashews in the mix and dehydrate overnight for 8–12 hours or until dry.

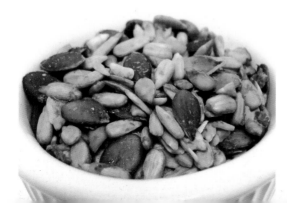
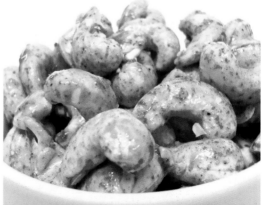

Pesto-stuffed Mushrooms

Marinate your mushrooms for at least 1 hour, overnight is best.

10 oz mushrooms
tamari sauce
olive oil

Destalk and marinate mushrooms in tamari sauce and olive oil for 1 hour. Dehydrate for 2 hours. Fill with basil pesto (see page 129).

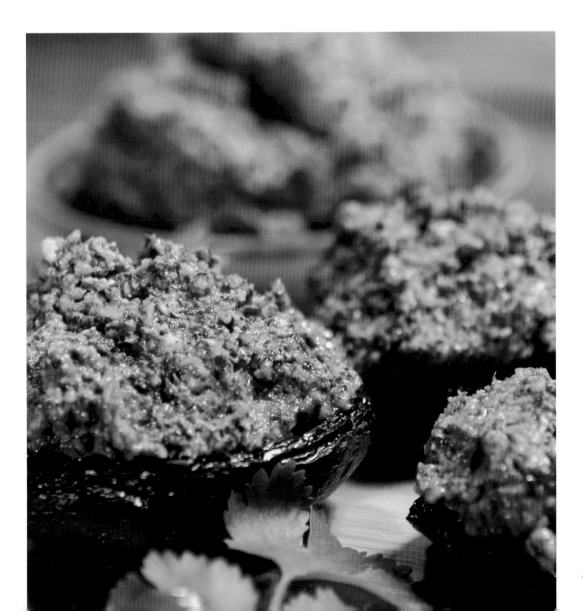

Broccoli Chips

This is one of the tastiest ways to eat raw broccoli. When we made this recipe for the first time Peter's brother told us it was his favorite thing we'd ever made! They taste like salty crispy vegetable potato chips.

1–2 heads broccoli
tamari sauce
apple cider vinegar

Take your head of broccoli and cut it into tiny florets. Place the florets in a bowl and coat well with tamari sauce and apple cider vinegar. Dehydrate for 24 hours. Once dehydrated, they store well in a glass jar.

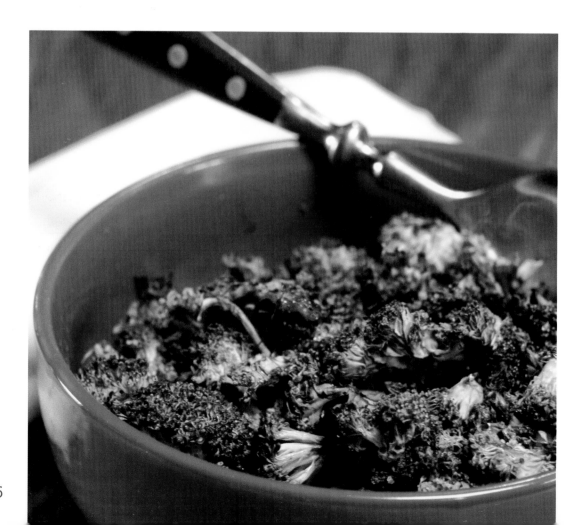

Eggplant Jerky

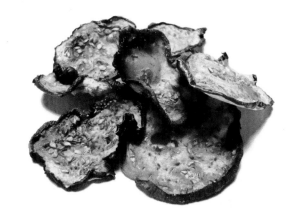

2 eggplants, sliced into thin rounds
⅓ cup (about 85 mL) apple cider vinegar
⅛ cup Bragg Liquid Aminos
¼ teaspoon Himalayan rock salt
¼ teaspoon cilantro powder
¼ teaspoon whole cilantro seeds
2 tablespoons tamari

Place the eggplants in a bowl and sprinkle with salt. Leave to stand and "sweat" for 1 hour. Drain and dry with a paper towel.
Make a marinade using the rest of the ingredients and press the eggplants into the marinade, almost bruising them slightly.
Place on a dehydrator sheet and dehydrate until crispy (approximately 12 hours).

Buckwheaties

4 cups (about 500 g) hulled buckwheat, soaked and sprouted
tamari sauce
Himalayan rock salt

For how to sprout buckwheat, see page 24.
When the buckwheat sprouts are ready place them in a bowl and coat lightly in tamari sauce and salt. Dehydrate them overnight (8–12 hours).

Buckwheaties are so nice! They add a crunch to salads, and can be sprinkled into soups as "croutons."

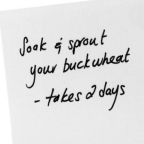

Soak & sprout
your buckwheat
– takes 2 days

Superfood Trail Mix

½ cup goji berries
½ cup cacao nibs
½ cup raisins
½ cup Brazil nuts
½ cup sunflower seeds
½ cup pumpkin seeds

Mix all the ingredients together in a large jar.

This little combination is a tasty weight-loss snack mix. It's super nutritious and will give your body true nourishment when you are hungry for a snack. Every time you feel the inclination to eat a sugary sweet muffin or a packet of potato chips, replace it with a handful or two of this superfood trail mix instead. Keep a pack in your handbag, on your desk, in your child's lunch box, and in your car.

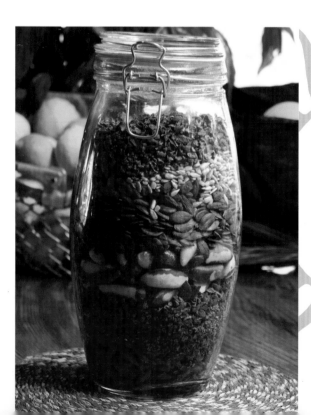

Goji berries are good for the immune system. Cacao nibs give you energy. Sunflower seeds are a good source of vitamin E. Pumpkin seeds are rich in omega oils. Brazil nuts reduce cancer risk.

Nutty Dates

pitted dates
pecans, walnuts, or cacao beans

Take the dates and open them slightly. Press the pecan, walnut, or cacao bean into the date. These make delicious travel snacks.

Dried Fruit

You can make your own preservative-free dried fruit using a dehydrator.

apples
pineapples
bananas
mangos
peaches
papaya

Take a selection of your favorite in-season fresh fruit, cut into slices or rings, and dehydrate until dry. Store in glass jars.

You can also make your own fruit rolls by making a sauce of your fresh fruit in a food processor or power blender and spreading the mixture out onto a solid dehydrator sheet and dehydrating until dry and flexible.

Dripping Dried Figs

This one is decadent!

dried figs
nut butter

Dip dried figs into your favorite nut butter and ENJOY!

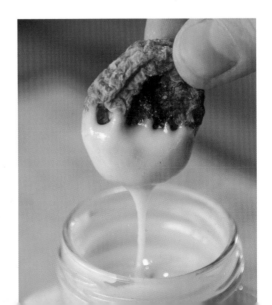

Cookies

Makes 20–30 cookies

Plain cookie base:
2 cups uncooked rolled oats
1 cup pitted dates, soaked
½ cup raisins
½ cup Brazil nuts
2 tablespoons honey

Soak the dates in some warm water for 10–15 minutes. The water should just cover the dates. In a food processor, grind up the oats and place in a mixing bowl. Coarsely chop the Brazil nuts and add to the mixing bowl along with the raisins. In the food processor or power blender blend the dates with half of the soak water until a jelly-like consistency is reached. Add the date jelly and honey to the mixing bowl and combine well. You may need to add some more date water to get a pliable consistency.

Once you've made the base mixture you can flavor your cookies in many ways. Here are some ideas:

Chocolate Cookies

Add 3–4 tablespoons cacao powder and a handful of cacao nibs.

Goji & Peach Cookies

Add a handful of goji berries and finely sliced dried peaches. You could also replace the date jelly with peach jelly for even more peachy-flavored cookies.

Apple, Raisin & Cinnamon Cookies

Add 1 chopped apple, 1 handful of chopped pecans, and 1 teaspoon of cinnamon.

Take the mixture and roll it into balls. Flatten them into round cookie shapes and place on a dehydrator tray. Dehydrate for 8–12 hours.

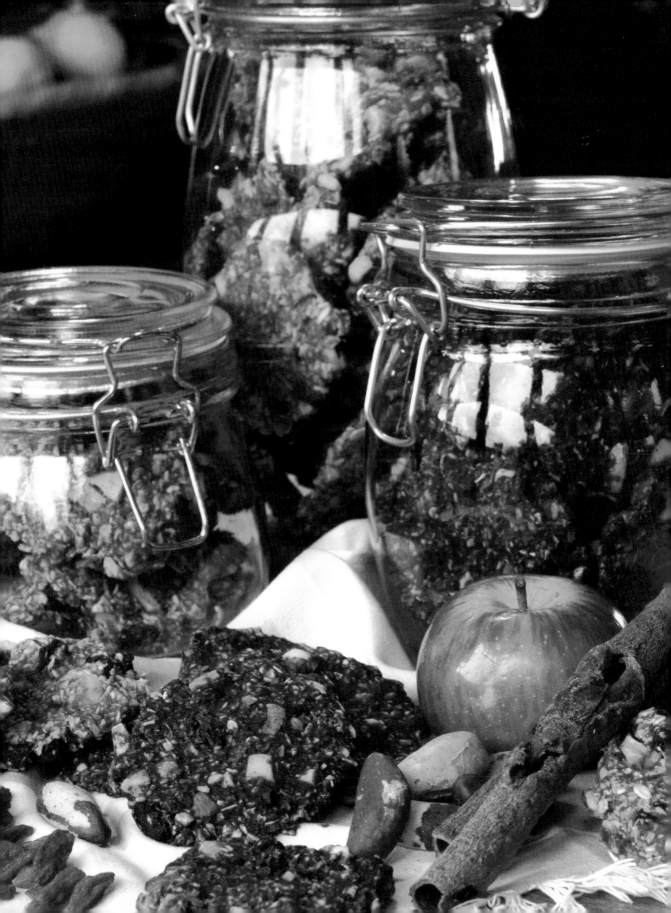

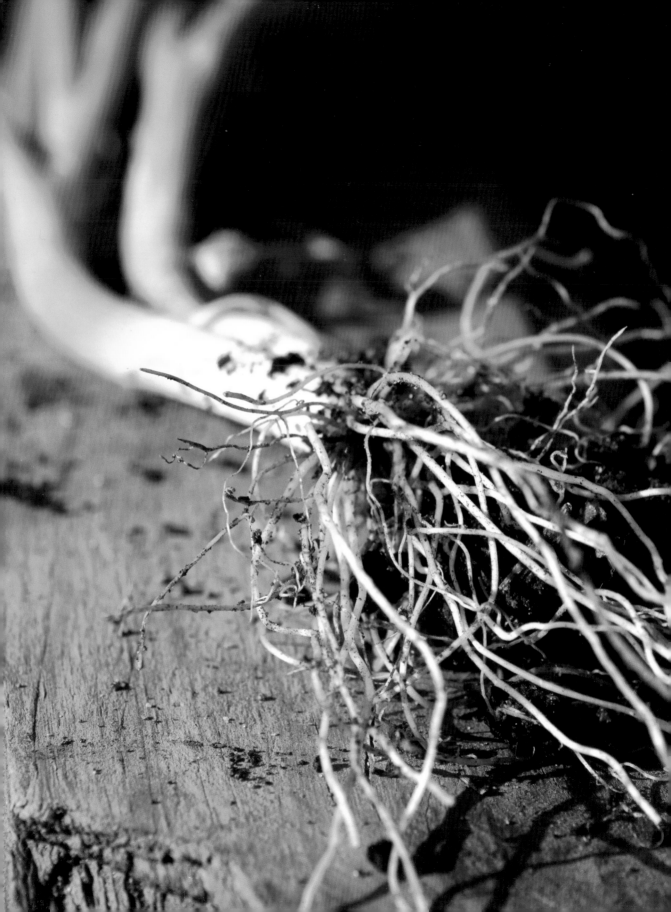

Simple Meals

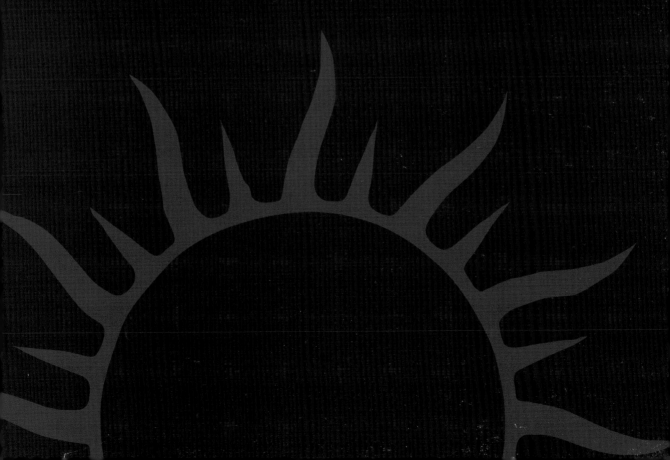

Leaf Wraps

If you want to make a really quick, simple meal that is really yummy, try this out.

1 large romaine or spinach leaf
1 avocado, sliced
½ tomato, diced
dried pitted dates or figs, chopped
Himalayan rock salt
tamari sauce

Use a big green leaf about the size of your hand (a large romaine lettuce leaf or spinach leaf works well). Prepare slices of avocado, diced tomato, and chopped dates or dried figs. Place the leaf on a plate and lay down the slices of avocado first, then the tomato, then the dried fruit. Add a pinch of salt and drizzle with tamari sauce. Roll up the edges and enjoy. This simple recipe is effective and surprisingly satisfying because it covers all three macronutrient food groups.

We've made many variations of this leaf wrap. Another good combo is using guacamole and olives as a filling. We were once given the biggest brassica leaves I've ever seen and made footlong leaf wraps with avocado, carrots, cucumber and turnip rice.

Turnip Rice

3–5 turnips, peeled
¼ cup macadamia nuts or pine nuts
1 tablespoon olive oil
2 tablespoons lemon juice
½ teaspoon Himalayan rock salt

Place all the ingredients in a food processor and blend until a ricelike consistency is reached.

You can make variations of this rice by using parsnips, white yams, or celeriac root.

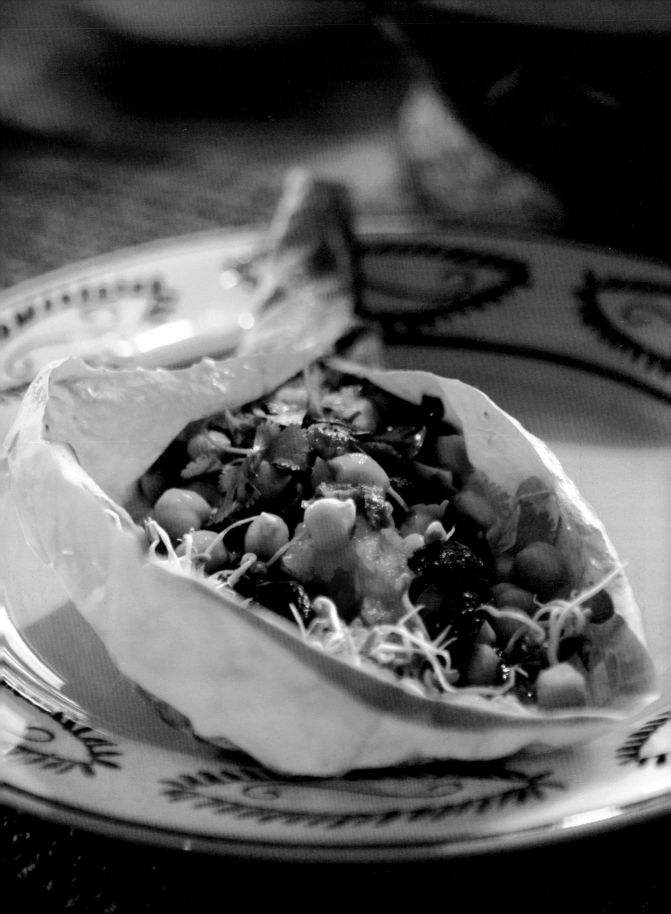

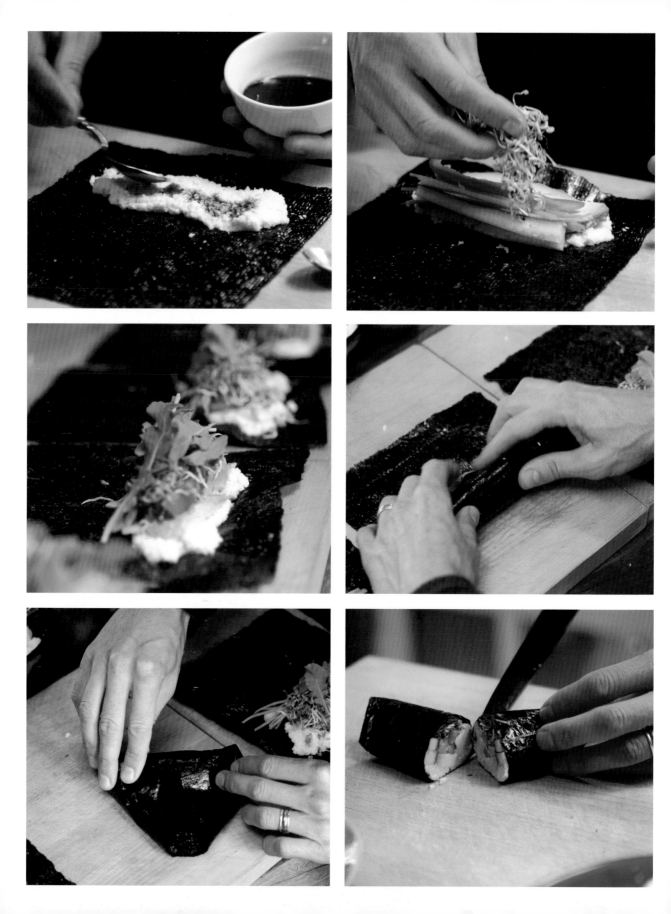

Sushi Handrolls

raw nori sheets
turnip rice
avocado slices
carrots, julienned
cucumber, julienned
red bell pepper, julienned
a selection of sprouts
arugula leaves
tamari sauce

Place a sushi sheet down on a chopping board. Place a layer of rice on the bottom half of the sushi nori sheet. Drizzle with tamari sauce. Layer the avocado, carrots, cucumber, and red bell pepper. Top with sprouts and arugula leaves and roll into a handroll by tucking in both ends and slicing in half.

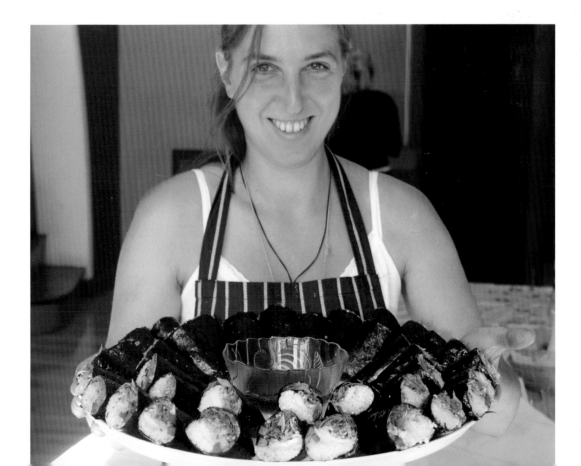

Marinated & Stuffed Red Bell Peppers

red bell peppers, cut in half and deseeded
olive oil
apple cider vinegar
Himalayan rock salt
creamed spinach
avocado, sliced
parsley to garnish

Take the halved and deseeded red bell peppers and place in a mixing bowl. Coat them in olive oil, apple cider vinegar, and salt. Place on a solid dehydrator sheet and dehydrate for 5–6 hours.

Make a batch of creamed spinach (see page 139) and stuff the bell peppers with this mixture. Top with slices of avocado, garnish with parsley, and serve.
Another stuffing alternative could be the sprouted quinoa salad (see page 121).

Meze Madness

My favorite way of entertaining is to have friends round for a meze meal. It's easy and quick to prepare all the sauces, dips, and salads plus it's a fun and interactive way of enjoying a meal together.
Here's how I do it.

Get a combination of dipping leaves, e.g., romaine, spinach, or sorrel leaves.

Prepare 2 or 3 dips such as:
Guacamole (see page 139)
Salsa (see page 139)
Pesto (see page 129)

MEZE
Choose your favourite combo of dips, sides, salads & dressings

Put out bowls of olives or buckwheaties.
Use the leaves instead of bread for dipping into these tasty spreads.

Make up a sprouted salad such as the sprouted chickpea salad (see page 123) and sushi handrolls (see page 157) for the real meze madness experience.

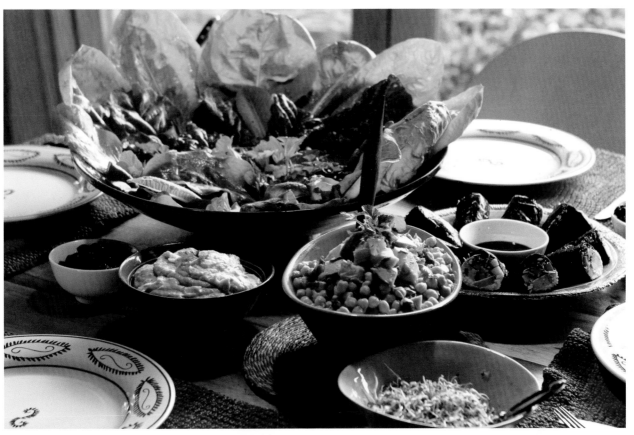

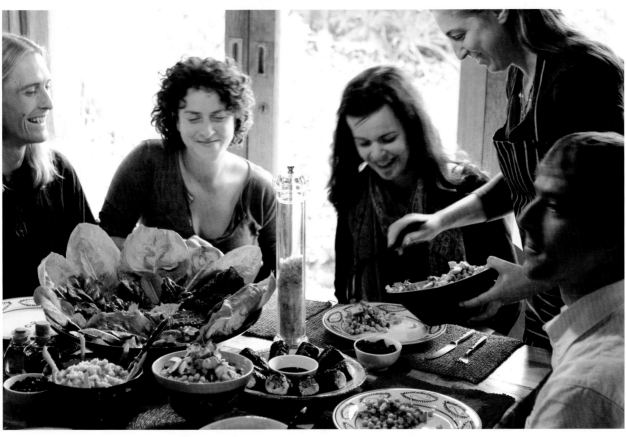

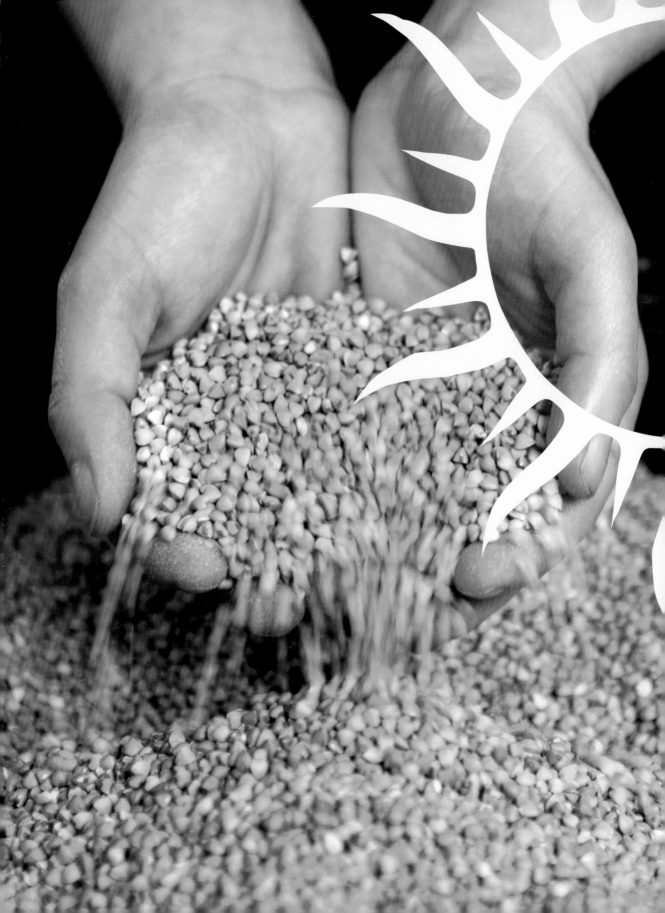

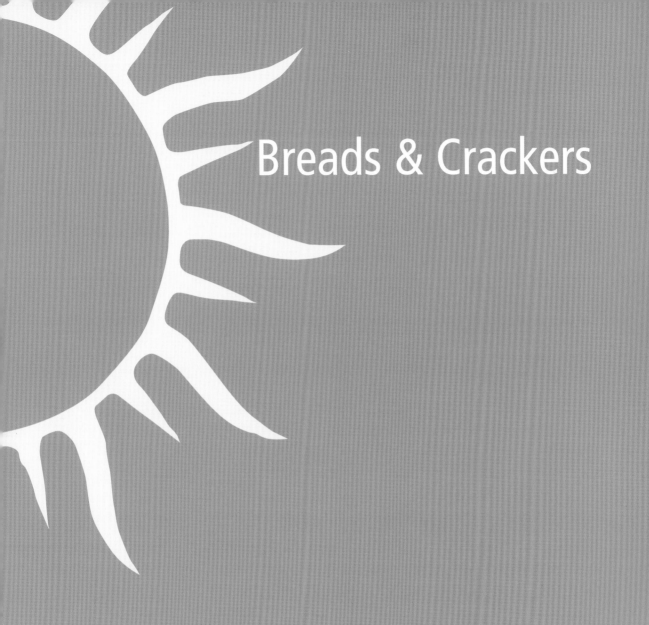

Breads & Crackers

One of the things that people find the hardest to give up when cutting out processed foods and switching to a higher raw plant-based diet are "foods" such as breads and crackers. Here are some raw, dehydrated options to get you over that hurdle.

Simple Flax Crackers

Plain Crackers

1 cup flaxseeds, ground
1 cup sunflower seeds
Juice of 1 lemon
½ teaspoon Himalayan rock salt
3 tablespoons olive oil
3 tablespoons tamari sauce

Process the flax and sunflower seeds in a food processor. Transfer this mixture into a mixing bowl and add lemon juice, salt, olive oil, and tamari sauce.

Press out the mixture onto solid dehydrator sheets. Use the lip of the dehydrator sheet as a gauge for thickness. Pressing out the mixture between two dehydrator sheets makes this process easier. Score the mixture into squares or wedges. Dehydrate overnight for 8–12 hours. In the morning turn the crackers out of the solid sheets and onto the mesh sheets and allow another 1–2 hours of drying time.

Create a variety of flavors by adding the following ingredients to the mixture:

Sundried Tomato and Olive Crackers

Add a handful of soaked and sliced sundried tomatoes and a handful of pitted and chopped olives.

Mixed Herb Crackers

Add ½ cup fresh chopped herbs such as thyme, oregano, and rosemary.

Flax-vegetable Crackers

2 cups golden flaxseeds, ground
5–6 zucchini, chopped
1 onion, chopped
1 clove garlic
1 tablespoon mixed herbs
⅛ cup olive oil
⅛ cup tamari
1 teaspoon Himalayan rock salt

Put all the ingredients into the food processor or power blender and process until smooth. Spread out onto solid dehydrator sheets. Score the mixture into squares or wedges and dehydrate overnight for 8–12 hours. In the morning turn the crackers out of the solid sheets and onto the mesh sheets and allow another 1–2 hours of drying time or until completely dry and crispy.

Flax is an amazing source of fiber, as well as omega-3 oils.

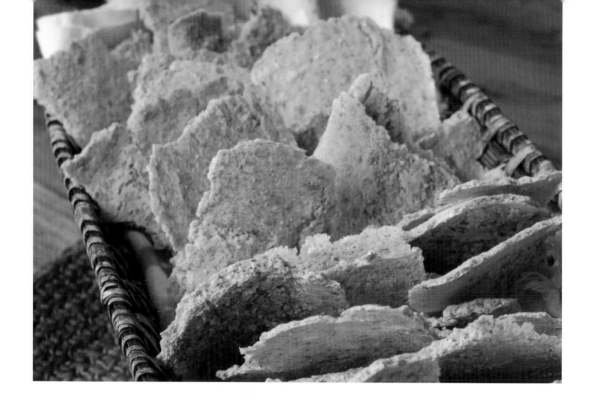

Buckwheat-flax Crackers

2 cups hulled buckwheat, soaked and sprouted
½ cup golden or brown flaxseeds, ground
⅓ cup flaxseeds, whole
2 tomatoes
1 yellow bell pepper
1 clove garlic
1 teaspoon Himalayan rock salt

Place all the ingredients in the food processor and mix until well combined. Spread the mixture out onto solid dehydrator sheets. Score the mixture into squares or wedges and dehydrate overnight for 8–12 hours. In the morning turn the crackers out of the solid sheets and onto the mesh sheets and allow another 1–2 hours of drying time or until completely dry and crispy.

Buckwheat is a fruit seed that is related to rhubarb and sorrel, making it suitable for people who are gluten sensitive. Its rich supply of flavonoids has been linked to lowered risk of high cholesterol and high blood pressure.

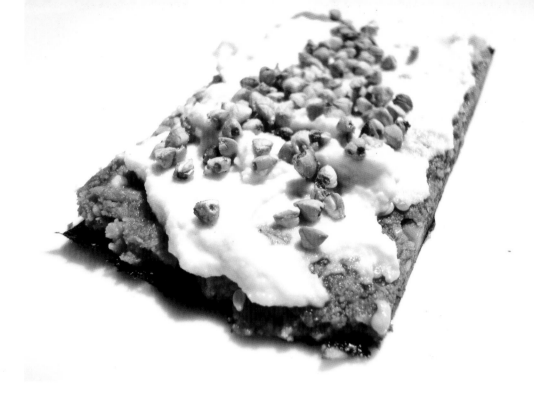

Nori Sesame Crackers

These are delicious, crumbly, and flavorful crackers with an Asian touch.
This is an adaptation of a nori cracker recipe in Rose Lee Calabro's book, *Living in the Raw Gourmet*, and is the outright cracker favorite in our household.

1 cup almonds, soaked overnight
1 cup walnuts, soaked for 2 hours
½ cup sunflower seeds, soaked for 2 hours
½ cup pumpkin seeds, soaked for 2 hours
¼ cup tahini
½ cup mixed fresh herbs, e.g., basil, thyme, rosemary, and oregano
1 clove garlic
2 tablespoons lemon juice
5 nori sheets
sesame seeds

Soak your nuts & seeds

In a food processor process all the ingredients excluding the nori sheets and sesame seeds. Spread the mixture thinly and evenly over the nori sheets using your hands to press it down, and a spatula to smooth it over. Sprinkle with sesame seeds and press them into the crackers. Score the mixture to desired shapes. Dehydrate for 12–24 hours or until the desired crispiness is reached. Store in an airtight container.

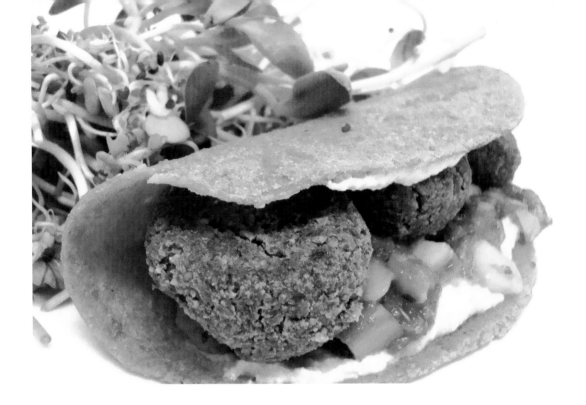

Sunshine Tortillas & Nachos

2 cups golden flaxseeds, ground
3 yellow bell peppers
¼ red onion
2 teaspoons Himalayan rock salt
1 tablespoon olive oil
1 teaspoon cumin seeds

Blend the yellow bell peppers, onion, salt, and olive oil in a power blender first. Then add the ground flax and cumin seeds and blend again using the tamper to make sure everything is well mixed through. Spread the batter over solid dehydrator sheets with a spatula and dehydrate for 2–3 hours. Turn out of the solid sheet and dehydrate for a further 1–2 hours, until a flexible tortilla consistency is reached. Cut into rounds and serve with hummus (see page 130), mango atchar (see page 140), and falafel balls (see page 179).

For nachos, score the mixture into squares or triangles and dehydrate overnight for 8–12 hours. In the morning turn the nachos out of the solid sheets and onto the mesh sheets. Allow another 1–2 hours of drying time or until completely dry and crispy. Serve with guacamole and salsa (see page 139).

Essene Bread

Unfortunately the wheat and bread products we see on the shelves of our supermarkets are mostly white and fluffy and bear no resemblance to the original whole wheat berry or wheat seed. Very often people find they are allergic to wheat because of its excessive processing and additives.

Essene bread is incredibly delicious. It is a moist and sweet bread. A dense bread with no yeast, sugar, preservatives, additives, or salt, it is made from 100 percent sprouted wheat seeds and is actually fairly simple to prepare.

Simple recipe

2 cups sprouted wheat seeds
2 tablespoons water
1 tablespoon olive oil
½ teaspoon mixed dried herbs
½ teaspoon Himalayan rock salt

Gourmet version

2 cups sprouted wheat seeds
½ apple
⅓ cup almonds, soaked for 30 minutes
⅓ cup walnuts, soaked for 30 minutes
⅓ cup (about 85 mL) olive oil
4 pitted dates, soaked for 30 minutes
2 tablespoons hemp seed protein powder
½ teaspoon Himalayan rock salt

Sprouting wheat increases the nutritional value of the grain and makes it easier to digest.

Sprout your wheat seeds (see page 24 for how to sprout wheat).
Grind the sprouted wheat seeds through the solid or flat-plate screen of a masticating juicer such as the Oscar. Alternatively, grind the seeds in a food processor. Place the ground seeds in the food processor with the remaining ingredients and process until a dough ball has formed. Using your hands, form the dough ball into a long flat loaf shape on a solid dehydrator sheet and flatten to approximately 4 inches (10 cm) long and ½–1 inch (1–2 cm) thick. Dehydrate for 12–24 hours. The outside should go crispy whilst the inside stays fairly moist. Cut into slices and serve.

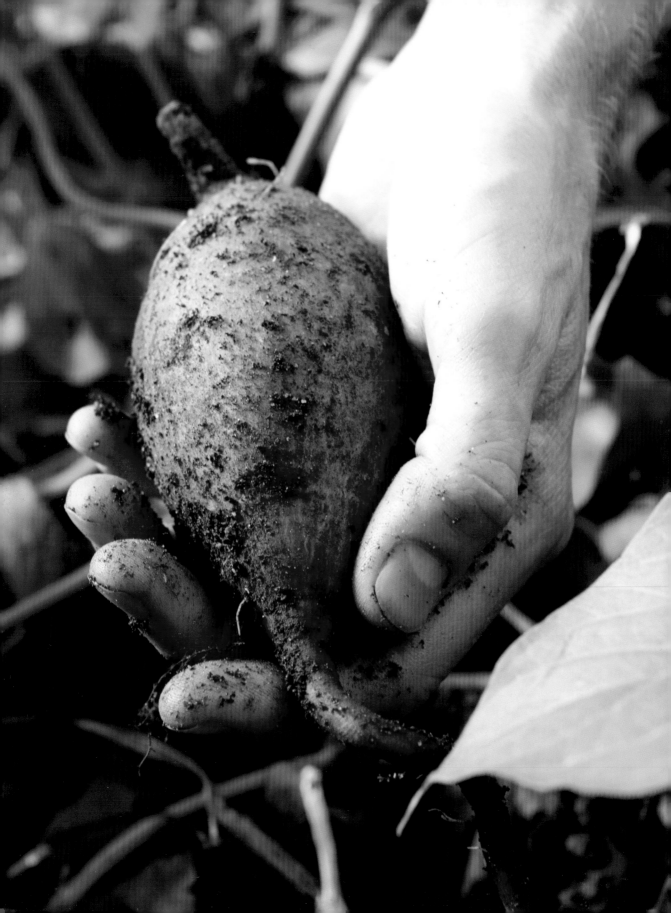

Gourmet Meals

Creamed Spinach & Mushroom Quiche

Red Bell Pepper, Tomato & Onion Quiche

Buckwheat Pizza

Yam – Pesto – Pasta

Butternut – Tomato – Pasta

Zucchini Pasta with Garlic White Sauce

Beet & Turnip Ravioli

Falafel

Lentil Burgers

Avocado Fouette with "Tuna" Mayo

These are the recipes with which you can impress your friends. In fact, invite them over, don't tell them you are serving only raw food, and see if they notice. These are raw versions of commonly cooked dishes. When I realized that eating raw food wasn't about depriving myself of the foods I used to love to eat but simply finding alternative ingredients and ways of preparing them, the doorway to a new healthy lifestyle was truly opened.

Some of these recipes can be time-consuming to prepare, especially when you take the dehydrating time into consideration, so plan ahead. On the other hand, some are really quick, such as the pastas. If you have batches of the different sauces already prepared these gourmet options won't seem overwhelming or out of reach. Remember, the first time you try something new it normally takes a bit more time, but by the second or third time around you'll be breezing.

Summer Quiches

Creamed Spinach & Mushroom Quiche

Makes 3–4 quiches

For the base:
1 cup almonds, soaked for 2 hours
½ cup flaxseeds, ground
2 zucchini, peeled and grated
¼ onion
2 teaspoons water
½ teaspoon Himalayan rock salt

In a food processor grind the almonds to a fine consistency. Add the ground flaxseeds, chopped onion, grated zucchini, water, and salt, and process until a light doughy consistency forms in the bowl. Make dough balls and place them on a solid dehydrator sheet. Press out into round bases and add a lip. Dehydrate for 2 hours. Remove from the solid sheet and dehydrate for another hour.

Creamed Spinach filling:
1 cup cashew nuts
¼ cup pine nuts
¾ cup water
¼ onion
½ teaspoon Himalayan rock salt
2 teaspoons nutritional yeast
4 cups baby spinach

Finely chop 4 cups of spinach. Process all the ingredients except 2 cups of chopped spinach in a food processor or power blender. Turn out the green-colored creamy sauce into a bowl and add the 2 remaining cups of spinach and stir through by hand.

Shiitake Mushrooms:
10 oz shiitake mushrooms

Slice the mushrooms and marinate in olive oil and tamari sauce for 1 hour.

Marinated Bell Peppers & Onions:
1 red bell pepper, sliced into strips
1 red onion, cut into rings
olive oil
honey

Marinate the red bell pepper slices and onion rings in olive oil and honey for 2 hours. Place on a solid sheet in the dehydrator and dehydrate for approximately 8 hours. The longer they dehydrate the nicer they taste.

Assembly:
Take your quiche base, fill it with the creamed spinach mixture, and place 5 slices of mushrooms over the filling. On a plate decorate with 3 slices of red bell pepper and top with onion rings.

Red Bell Pepper, Tomato & Onion Quiche

Makes 3–4 quiches

For the base:
1 cup almonds, soaked for 2 hours
2 small zucchini, peeled
½ cup buckwheat, soaked & sprouted
2 tablespoons flax meal
½ red onion
1 clove garlic
1 tablespoon lemon juice
2 teaspoons olive oil
½ teaspoon Himalayan rock salt

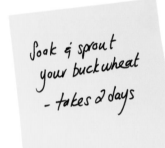

Soak & sprout your buckwheat – takes 2 days

Place all the ingredients in a food processor and blend into a doughy consistency. Place on a solid dehydrator sheet and press out into quiche shapes or press into miniature quiche tartlet tins (lined with plastic wrap). Dehydrate overnight for 12–14 hours.

Red Bell Pepper & Tomato filling:
1 red bell pepper
1 tomato
¼ cup cashew nuts
¼ cup sundried tomatoes, soaked
⅛ cup pitted olives
¼ red onion
½ garlic clove
1 tablespoon parsley, chopped
1 tablespoon basil, chopped
1 tablespoon lemon juice
1 tablespoon olive oil

For the garnish:
1 tomato, sliced thinly
4 sprigs of parsley
marinated onions (see page 141)

In a power blender combine all the ingredients and blend until smooth. Take the quiche bases out of the dehydrator and fill with this mixture. Top with tomato slices and dehydrate for a further 6 hours. Top with marinated onions and a sprig of parsley.

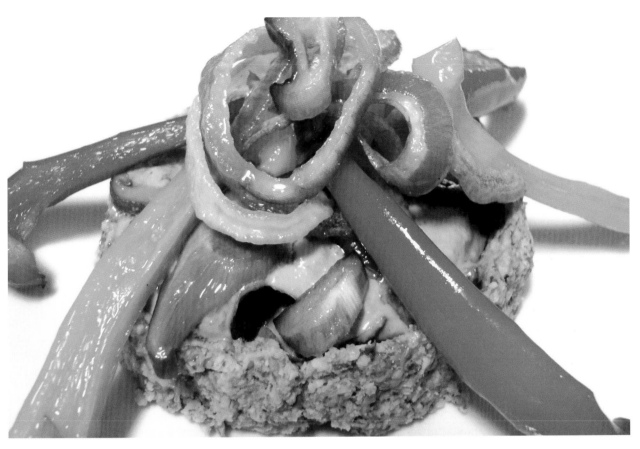

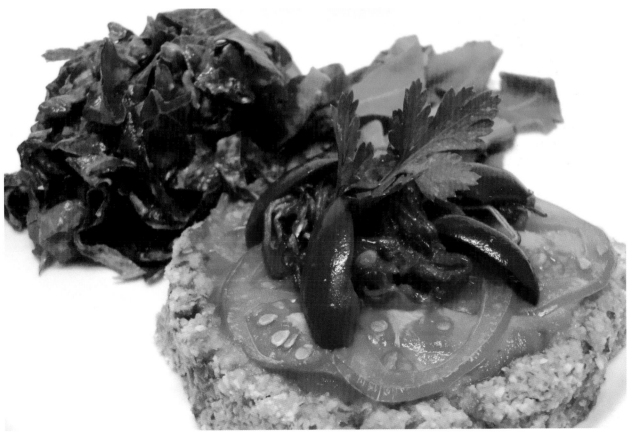

Pizza, Pasta & Ravioli

Buckwheat Pizza

For the crust:
2 cups hulled buckwheat, soaked and sprouted
1½ cups golden or brown flaxseeds, ground
6 zucchini, peeled
2 tomatoes
½ red onion
⅛ cups tamari sauce
¼ cup (about 65 mL) olive oil
1 clove garlic
1 teaspoon Himalayan rock salt

Place all the ingredients in the food processor and mix until well combined. Spread the mixture out onto solid dehydrator sheets. Dehydrate overnight for 8 – 12 hours. In the morning turn the pizza crust out of the solid sheets and onto the mesh sheets and allow another 1–2 hours of drying time. Makes three crusts.

Tomato sauce (see page 129)

For the toppings:
finely chopped spinach
baby tomatoes
red bell peppers
pitted olives

Instant Cashew Nut Cheese (see page 82)

Once you have dehydrated your pizza crust, spread the tomato sauce over the base. Top with your favorite toppings. Make a batch of instant cashew nut cheese and pour over the top. Dehydrate with all the toppings for a further 45 minutes to 1 hour.

Make your pizza crust, tomato sauce & nut cheese in advance.

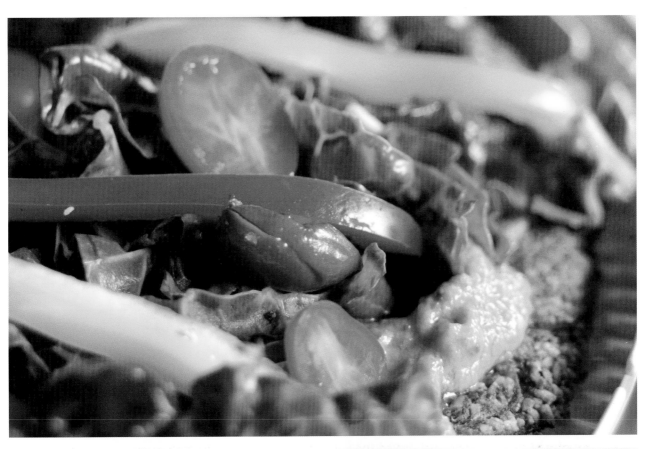

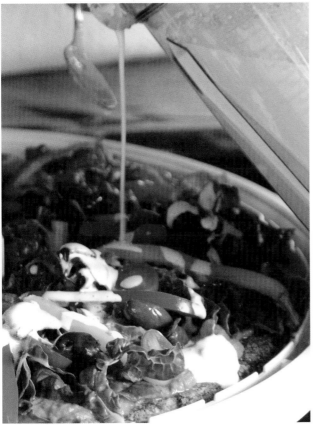

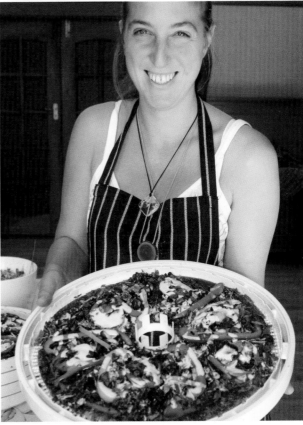

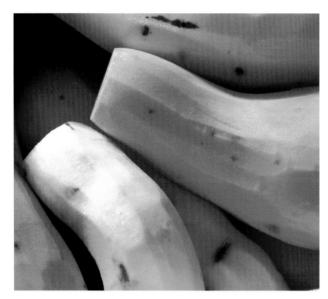
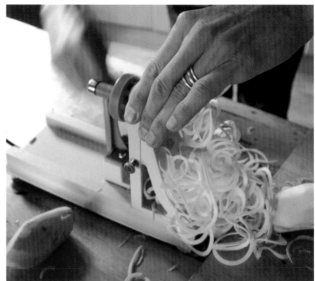
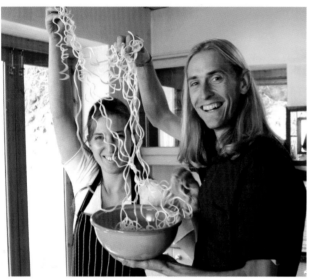
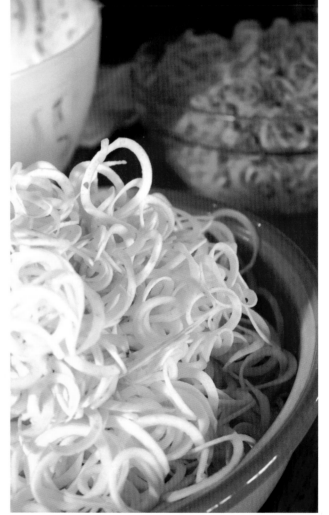
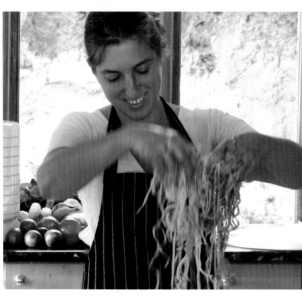

Pasta

Here you will need a kitchen tool called a spiralizer. With this little tool you can make pasta noodles in minutes.

The best vegetables to use are root veggies such as yam, butternut squash, turnip, and zucchini. The spiralizer comes with three different attachments for creating differently shaped noodles, so play with them and see which shapes you like the best.

The alternative to spiralizing your vegetables is to use a mandolin. Adjust the mandolin to a very thin setting and slice the zucchini into strips. A simple peeler can also do a great job of turning zucchini into tagliatelli-style strips or zucchini pasta.

These are the vegetable-sauce combinations that we like the most:

Yam – Pesto – Pasta

Yams, washed, peeled, and spiralized

Make up a batch of basil pesto (see page 129).
Mix the pesto through with your yam noodles.

Butternut – Tomato – Pasta

Butternut squash, peeled and spiralized

Make up a batch of tomato sauce (see page 129).
Mix the tomato sauce through with your butternut noodles.

Yams have far higher levels of nutrients than their poisonous cousin, the normal potato. They have significant antioxidant capacities. They are also an excellent source of vitamin A, vitamin C, and manganese.

Zucchini Pasta with Garlic White Sauce

Zucchini, peeled and spiralized or mandolined

Make up a batch of garlic white sauce (see page 131).
Mix the garlic and white sauce through with your zucchini noodles or zucchini pasta strips.

Beet & Turnip Ravioli

beet
turnips
cream cheese (see page 82)
spinach, finely chopped
garlic white sauce (see page 131)
scallions

Using a mandolin, cut very thin rounds of beets and turnips. Salt the slices and allow them to "sweat" for 10 minutes. Take your cream cheese and combine it with some finely chopped spinach. Take a beet or turnip round, put a dollop of cream cheese with spinach in the middle, and close it over with another round. Dehydrate for 2–3 hours.

Make a batch of garlic white sauce in your power blender and leave it running in the blender until slightly warmed. Place the warmed garlic sauce in a bowl and serve the ravioli on top of the warm sauce garnished with scallions.

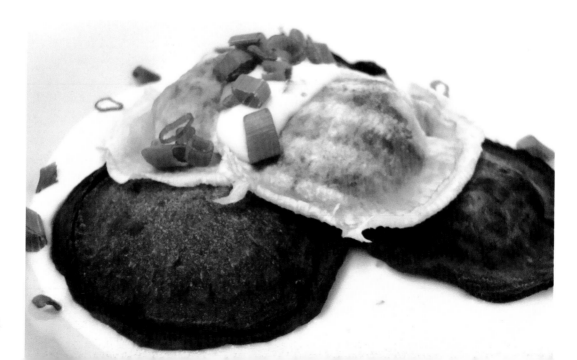

Falafel

Makes 24

1 cup chickpeas, sprouted
1 cup sunflower seeds
½ cup almonds, soaked for 2 hours
½ cup walnuts, soaked for 2 hours
¼ onion
¼ cup parsley, chopped
¼ cup cilantro, chopped
2 cloves garlic
2 tablespoons olive oil
2 tablespoons lemon juice
¼ cup tamari
1 teaspoon Himalayan rock salt
½ teaspoon black pepper

Sprout your chickpeas & soak the almonds, walnuts and sunflower seeds.

In a food processor finely grind the first four ingredients. Add the rest of the ingredients and blend again. Roll into balls and place on a solid dehydrator tray. Dehydrate for 12 hours. Serve in a sunshine tortilla (see page 166) with hummus (see page 130), salsa (see page 139), and a salad.

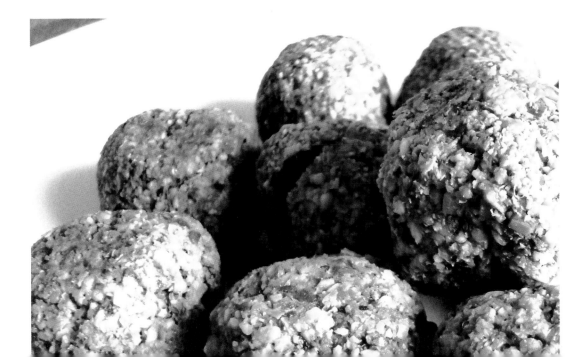

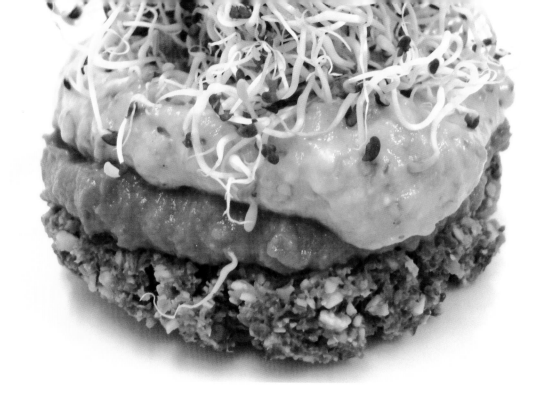

Lentil Burgers

2 cups walnuts, soaked for 2 hours
2 cups sprouted lentils
2 large carrots, peeled and grated
1 large onion
2 cloves garlic
¼ cup (about 65 mL) Bragg Liquid Aminos
¼ cup (about 65 mL) olive oil
½ cup parsley, chopped
1 teaspoon Himalayan rock salt

Combine all the ingredients together in a food processor. Shape into patties and place in the dehydrator to dry for 12–14 hours.

Soak walnuts and sprout lentils.

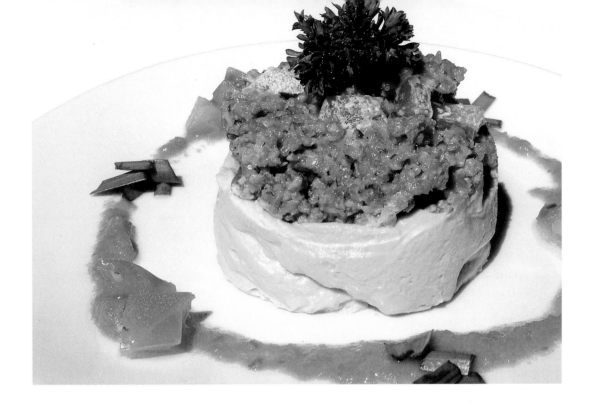

Avocado Fouette with "Tuna" Mayo

Makes 6

½ cup cashew nuts
⅛ cup coconut oil
½ garlic clove
1 teaspoon Himalayan rock salt
2 avocados
1 teaspoon Bragg Liquid Aminos
½ tablespoon olive oil
Juice of half a lemon
"Tuna" Mayo (see page 125)

Blend the cashews and coconut oil in the power blender until smooth.
Add the remaining ingredients and blend again.
Place the mixture in a mousse ring lined with wax paper and refrigerate. Make up
a batch of the "Tuna" mayo. Take the avocado base out of the refrigerator, gently
remove the mousse ring, and peel away the wax paper. Top with the "Tuna" mayo.
Serve with a bed of arugula and sprouts and garnish with parsley.

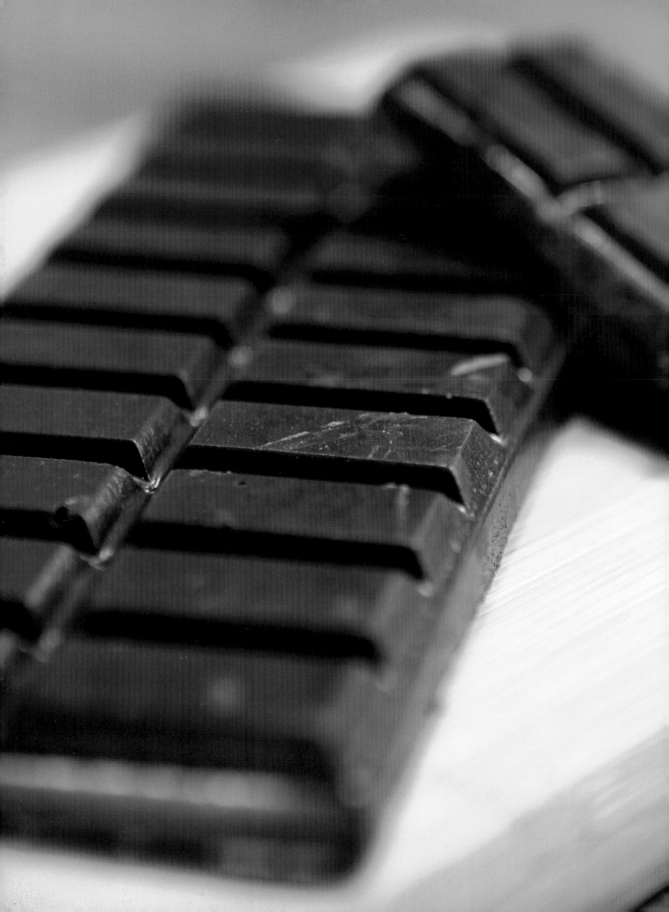

Healthy Desserts

Apple Tart with Mango Custard

Mango Tart

Lemon Tart

Mango-gooseberry Cheesecake

Chocolate Love Cake

Vanilla-maple Ice Cream

Chocolate Sauce

Creamy Banana & Cashew Ice Cream

Heavenly Fruit with Sweet Nut Cream

Chocolate Brownies

Chocolate Mousse

Mint-choc Discs

Chocolates

This is undoubtedly my favorite section. "Healthy" and "desserts" are two words that I used to think were mutually exclusive. I am always happy to admit that I entered the world of raw foods via my taste buds and the back door of sweet treats. I never woke up one day and said, "I must get healthy, it's time to go raw." I tasted a raw food cake and said, "Mmmmm, this tastes good – I can do more of this."

Cakes & Tarts

Apple Tart with Mango Custard

I make this cake using the solid dehydrator sheet as the cake base. You can also make small apple tartlets using mini quiche tins.

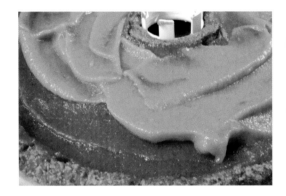
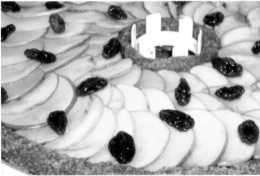

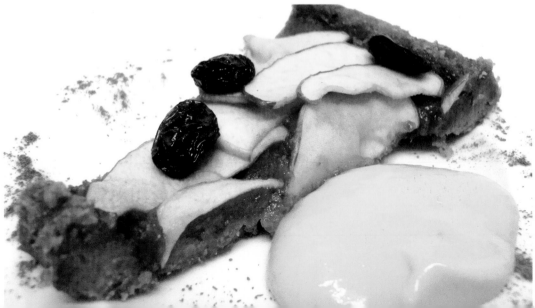

For the base:
3 cups walnuts, soaked for 2 hours
1 apple
2 zucchini
⅓ cup honey
Seeds of 1 vanilla pod

Make the base of this tart the day before – dehydrates overnight

Place the ingredients in a food processor, blend, and press out onto a solid dehydrator sheet. Dehydrate overnight for 8–12 hours.

Fig or Date Jelly:
1 cup figs or pitted dates, soaked

Blend the figs with some of the soak water in a power blender or food processor.

Apple Puree:
3 apples, peeled and cored
½ teaspoon ground cinnamon

Blend the apples in the food processor with the cinnamon.

Apple topping:
10 apples, finely sliced
¼ cup raisins
1 cup honey with 4 tablespoons hot water
1 tablespoon ground cinnamon
Juice of 1 lemon

Soak the apples and raisins in the honey-cinnamon-water mixture for 2–3 hours.

Assembly:
Take the dehydrated base and spread the fig or date jelly evenly over the base. Spread a layer of applesauce over the jelly.
Top with the sliced apples and sprinkle with raisins. Dehydrate for a further 2–3 hours.
Cut into slices and serve with a dollop of mango custard.

Mango Custard:
2–3 mangos
⅛ cup coconut oil, melted

Blend the ingredients together in a power blender and serve with the apple tart.

There are many fruit-based refrigerator tarts that you can make using raw ingredients. You simply mix up a base of nuts, seeds, or coconut flakes and then make a filling out of your favorite fruits combined with raw organic coconut oil. The key is in the coconut oil. Coconut oil is liquid at temperatures above 78.8°F and below 78.8°F it is solid. You can get just about any kind of coconut oil–based fruit tart to set in the refrigerator once you know this little secret.

Mango Tart

For the crust:
1½ cups cashews or almonds
3 cups shredded coconut
1 tablespoon lemon juice
Seeds of ½ vanilla pod
½ cup honey
1 tablespoon coconut oil

In a food processor grind the nuts into a fine crumb mixture.
Add the shredded coconut and the other remaining ingredients, and pulse until well combined. Use a quiche tin with removable base or a springform cake tin and press the mixture into the bottom. Make puncture holes in the base using a fork and put it into the refrigerator while you make the filling.

For the mango mousse filling:
5 ripe mangos
1 cup (250 mL) coconut oil
Seeds of ½ vanilla pod
½ teaspoon Himalayan rock salt

Blend all the ingredients together in a power blender. Get your base out of the refrigerator and pour the filling into the crust and refrigerate. Will set in 1–2 hours.

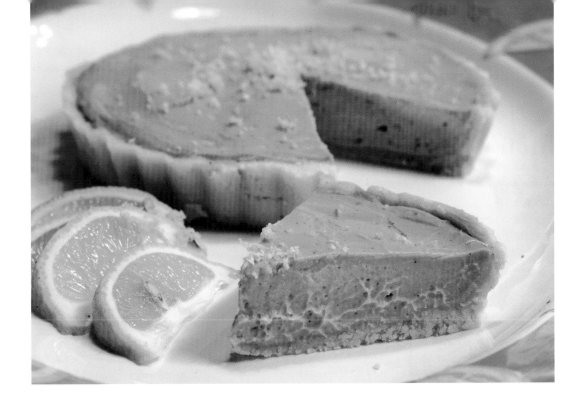

Lemon Tart

The first time I made this, Peter's mom thought I was making guacamole because of the green color. Peter's dad loves lemon-flavored desserts and they were both astonished when they tasted this avocado-based, sweet lemon tart.

Make up the same crust as the Mango Tart (see page 186)

For the lemon filling:
5 ripe avocados
¾ cup lemon juice
2 tablespoons lemon zest
¾ cup honey
1 cup (250 mL) coconut oil
Seeds of 1 vanilla pod
½ teaspoon Himalayan rock salt

Blend all the ingredients together in a power blender until smooth. Pour into the crust base and refrigerate.

In this recipe the avocados provide the bulk for the filling. The key with this tart is to put in enough lemon and honey to offset the flavor of the avocados.

Mango-gooseberry Cheesecake

In South Africa we are blessed with an abundant supply of mangos and gooseberries in summer.

For the base:
1 cup almonds, soaked for 2 hours
1 cup pecans, soaked for 2 hours
1 tablespoon honey
1 tablespoon coconut oil
Seeds of 1 vanilla pod
¼ teaspoon Himalayan salt
2 teaspoons lemon juice
3 tablespoons cacao powder

Put all the ingredients into a food processor and blend until finely chopped. Press into the base of a springform cake tin, make puncture holes in the base using a fork, and put it into the refrigerator while you make the filling.

For the filling:
2 cups cashew nuts
1 cup macadamia nuts
1 cup (250 mL) coconut oil
½ cup agave
¼ cup (about 65 mL) lemon juice
1–2 mangos
Seeds of 2 vanilla pods

For the topping:
6 passion fruit
1 cup raspberries
¼ cup agave

Cape gooseberries (also known as Incan or golden berries) are one of the top superfoods. They are extremely high in protein as well as phosphorous and vitamins A, C, B1, B2, and are one of the best sources of B6.

Blend all the ingredients for the filling together in a power blender until smooth. Make a double batch if you want a really tall cake. Pour the filling over the base. Make a passion fruit topping by putting the passion fruit into a bowl with agave nectar. Strain the excess liquid off the passion fruit and pour over the filling. Decorate with gooseberries and raspberries. Refrigerate overnight or place in the freezer to set.

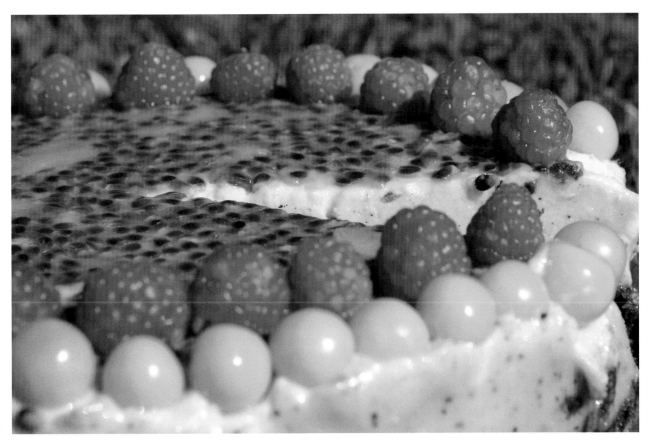

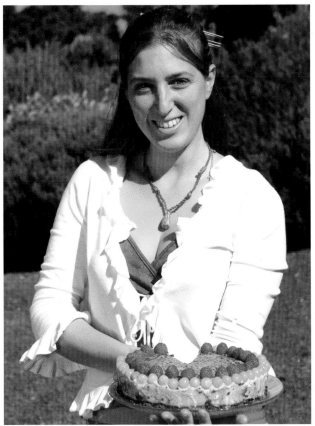

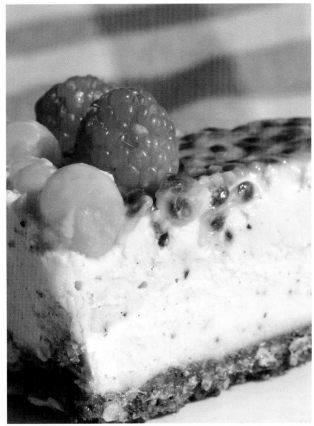

Chocolate Love Cake

For the base:
3 cups almonds, soaked for 2 hours
1 cup pecan nuts, soaked for 2 hours
¼ cup agave
Seeds of 2 vanilla pods
½ teaspoon Himalayan rock salt

In a food processor, grind the almonds and pecan nuts until fine. Add the agave, vanilla seeds, and salt. Process all the ingredients together until a sticky, crumble-like base is formed. You may need to stop and scrape down the sides. Press into a springform cake tin or quiche tin with removable base. Make puncture holes in the base using a fork and put it in the refrigerator while you make the topping.

For the topping:
4 cups pitted dates, soaked in warm water
1½ cups (375 mL) coconut oil
1 cup cacao powder
1 avocado
Seeds of 1 vanilla pod
1 teaspoon Himalayan rock salt

For decoration:
10 cacao beans
10 pecans

Blend the dates with a little of the soak water in a power blender or food processor. Add the coconut oil, cacao powder, vanilla seeds, avocado, and salt. Blend until all ingredients are mixed through. Transfer into the cake or quiche tin and spread evenly. Decorate with cacao beans and pecan nuts. Refrigerate for at least 1 hour.

The magnesium in cacao supports heart health and the good brain chemicals in chocolate make you feel blissful, which is why chocolate has always been associated with love.

Ice cream

There are many ways to make raw fruit or nut-based ice creams. The main ingredients for ice cream are nonperishable, so you can always have the items you need ready and waiting to go. It's a good idea to keep your cupboard well stocked with cashew or macadamia nuts and coconut oil. Keep peeled and frozen bananas in the freezer.

Vanilla-maple Ice cream

2 cups (500 mL) almond milk (see page 78)
1 cup macadamia nuts
½ cup maple syrup
Seeds of 2 vanilla pods
Pecan nuts, chopped (optional)

Needs to freeze overnight.

Blend all the ingredients together in a power blender until smooth.
Stir in chopped pecan nuts if you would like a maple-pecan nut version of this ice cream. Put the mixture in the freezer overnight to set. In the morning take the ice cream out of the freezer, slice it up, and process through the crushing screen of a masticating juicer such as the Oscar to remove the ice crystals. Refreeze or serve straight away. Beware of maple-flavored syrups.

Chocolate Sauce

⅓ cup (about 85 mL) coconut oil, melted
¼ cup maple syrup
¼ cup cacao powder

On low speed in a blender mix all the ingredients together or simply place the ingredients in a bowl and whisk with a fork.

Get out your ice cream, pour this chocolate sauce over it, and indulge guilt-free.

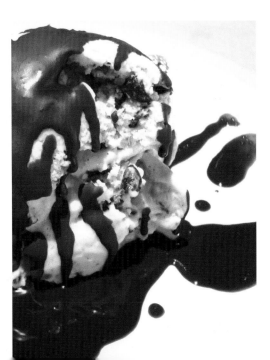

Creamy Banana & Cashew Ice Cream

2 cups cashew nuts
¾ cup coconut oil, melted
3 tablespoons honey
Seeds of 1 vanilla pod
4–5 frozen bananas
A little water

Blend the cashews, honey, coconut oil, and vanilla seeds in a power blender until a smooth, creamy consistency is reached. Blend the frozen bananas in the food processor with a little bit of water until it resembles a smooth, soft-serve ice cream. Slowly pour the blended cashew mix into the food processor as it is turning, until a fluffy, creamy consistency is reached. Place in the freezer to set for 2 hours.

Other Variations

Once we discovered how delicious this ice cream was we started to experiment with different flavors. Peter and I both jumped into the kitchen and within an hour we had choc-chip, mint-choc-chip, and chocolate mint-choc-chip versions.

Choc-chip:
Add cacao nibs to the base mixture, stir through, and set.

Mint choc-chop:
Add a drop of organic mint essential oil to the choc-chip version above.

Chocolate mint-choc-chip:
Add 1–2 tablespoons cacao powder to the mint choc-chip version above.

Strawberry:
Add 2 cups strawberries to the original banana-cashew mixture.

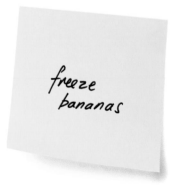

freeze
bananas

Dessert in a Glass

Heavenly Fruit with Sweet Nut Cream

For the fruit part:
A selection of seasonal fruit of your choice such as berries, mangos, peaches, passion fruit, guavas, papayas, bananas, and pomegranates.

For the sweet nut cream:
3 cups macadamia nuts
1 cup (250 mL) freshly squeezed orange or clementine juice
2 tablespoons honey
A sprig of mint for each glass

Place a layer of fruit in an attractive glass. Add a layer of cream. Place another layer of fruit on top of the cream layer. Continue like this until the glass is full, ending with a delectable whirl of cream and a sprig of fresh mint.

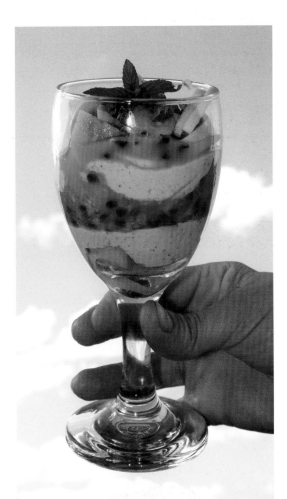

Chocolate Indulgence

Chocolate Brownies

2 cups almonds, soaked for 2 hours
1½ cups cacao powder
¼ cup maple syrup
⅛ cup agave
½ cup (125 mL) water
Seeds of 1 vanilla pod
½ avocado
¼ teaspoon ground cinnamon
¼ teaspoon Himalayan rock salt
Wax paper

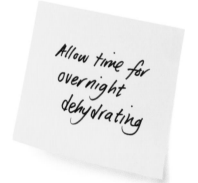

Allow time for overnight dehydrating

Crush the almonds by putting them through the solid plate or crushing screen of a masticating juicer. Put the finely crushed almonds into a food processor with the remaining ingredients and combine well. Press the mixture out onto strips of wax paper and fold up the edges to hold the brownies in shape. Dehydrate for 14 hours. Slice and serve with chocolate sauce (see page 191), a sweet nut cream (see page 193), and gooseberries.

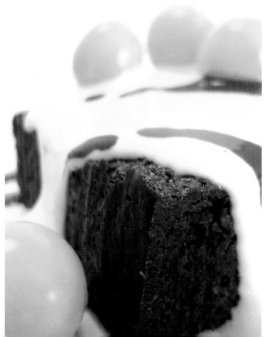

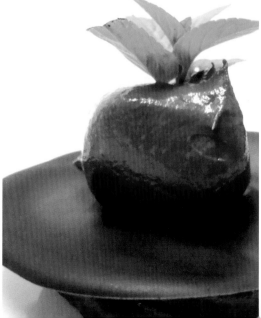

Chocolate Mousse

This is another avocado dessert special. It stores unbelievably well for up to a week in the refrigerator, even though you would think that the avocados should brown or start to taste funny after a few days. As with the lemon tart, the key is to add enough sweetness to offset the taste of the avocados and enough cacao powder to change the color.

4 avocados
1 cup cacao powder
¼ cup (about 65 mL) coconut oil
½–¾ cup maple syrup
¼ cup (about 65 mL) water

Blend all the ingredients in a power blender until smooth.
For a real gourmet presentation, make the Mint-choc Discs (see below).

Mint-choc Discs

Makes 20

7 oz (200g) cacao butter, melted
½ cup cacao powder
¼ cup maple syrup
1 drop mint essential oil
Wax paper

Melt the cacao butter in a double boiler or over a pot of water at low temperature. Once melted, put all the ingredients into a blender and mix on low speed until everything is well combined. Place a large spoonful of the chocolate mixture onto a sheet of wax paper. Using the back of a spoon spread the mixture into thin disc shapes. Place in the freezer to set.

For a gourmet presentation of the chocolate mousse, put 1 large dollop of chocolate mousse in the middle of a plate. Gently peel 1 chocolate disc away from the wax paper and place it on top of the chocolate mousse. Add another dollop on top of the chocolate disc and top with a mint leaf. Dust the plate with cacao powder or for full indulgence, drizzle with chocolate sauce. You can even make a double choc-disc tower!

Chocolates

Plain Chocolates

7 oz (200 g) cacao butter, melted
½ cup (125 mL) coconut oil, melted
½ cup agave
2 cups cacao powder
Seeds of 1 vanilla pod

Melt the cacao butter in a double boiler or over a pot of water at low temperature. Put the melted liquid into your power blender. Add the melted coconut oil, agave, and vanilla seeds and blend. Slowly sieve the cacao powder into the mixture and blend on low speed until everything is combined. All the ingredients can be mixed through by hand if you do not have a power blender.

Pour into chocolate molds or ice trays and allow to set in the refrigerator.

Other flavors

Nutty Chocs:
Add a handful of your favorite chopped nuts into your chocolate mixture and set.

Fruity Chocs:
Add a handful of raisins or goji berries to your chocolate mixture and set.

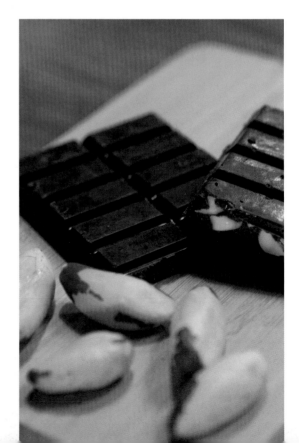

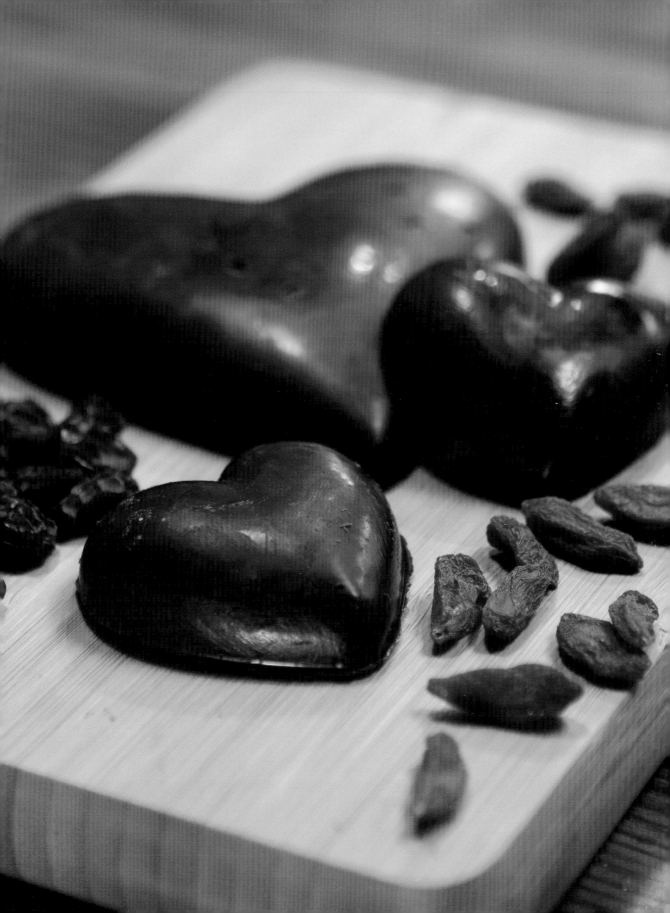

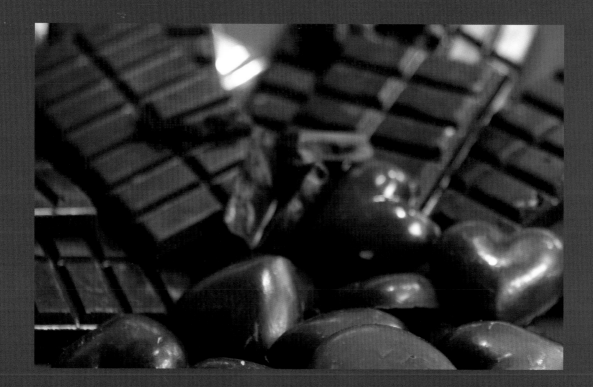

Ashwagandha Perhaps the most famous adaptogenic Ayurvedic herb, it boosts the immune system and reduces stress.

Astragalus Used in traditional Chinese medicine to support and enhance the immune system.

Sceletium Revered shrub of the San people. Sceletium elevates the mood and decreases anxiety, stress, and tension, as well as being an effective antidepressant.

Ginseng Has a powerful ability to restore vigor, increase longevity, enhance overall health, and stimulate both a healthy appetite and a good memory.

Taheebo One of the world's most powerful herbs. Also called Pau d'Arco, it has strong antifungal and antibiotic properties.

Foti In China, Foti is known as Ho Shou Wu and has a reputation for enhancing longevity and energy, and serving as a tonic to increase overall vitality.

Cat's Claw Miracle herb from the rain forests of Peru. Its antiviral and anti-inflammatory properties enhance the immune system and gastro-intestinal tract.

Medicinal Chocolates

The most healing way of eating chocolate is to use cacao as a carrier of medicine. The medicine will be in the form of herbs and spices added to the chocolate mixture. Cacao has a natural ability to allow the body to absorb more of the healing qualities of herbs.

9 oz (250g) cacao butter, melted
¼ cup (about 65 mL) coconut oil
4 tablespoons honey
2 cups cacao powder
½ teaspoon ashwagandha
1 teaspoon astragalus
⅛ teaspoon sceletium
¼ teaspoon red ginseng
½ teaspoon taheebo
¼ teaspoon cat's claw
½ teaspoon Siberian ginseng
1½ teaspoons buchu powder or sprig of fresh mint
½ tablespoon maca
1 tablespoon foti
½ teaspoon cayenne pepper

Melt the cacao butter in a double boiler or over a pot of water at low temperature. Put the melted liquid into your power blender. Add the melted coconut oil and honey and blend. Slowly sieve the cacao powder into the liquid mixture, blending on low speed. Add the herbs and continue to blend until everything is mixed through.

Pour into chocolate molds or ice trays and allow to set in the refrigerator.

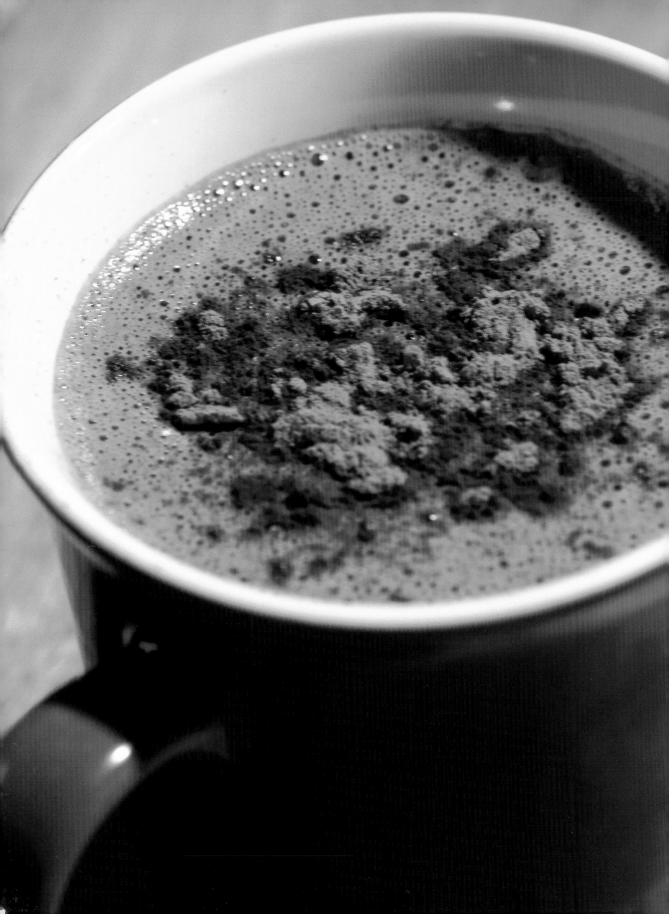

Other Beverages

Herbal Infusions

Iced Frappacino

Lexi's Cuppa Chai

Mint-coca-sesame Tea

Coff-tea

Hot Chocolate

Cold Beverages

Herbal Infusions

For an uplifting variation, infuse and flavor your drinking water with the following herbs.

Put 2 cups (500 mL) fresh spring water in a bottle or jar and allow to infuse for 3–4 hours with the following combination of ingredients.

Cinnamon and bay leaves
Lavender, rosemary, and ginger
Buchu or mint
Mint and geranium
Goji berries and a vanilla pod

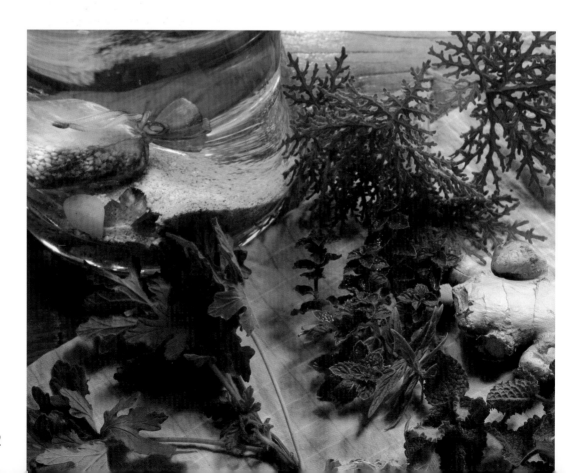

Iced Frappacino

Makes 3–4 glasses

This drink has a dark, chocolatey flavor and a stimulating coffee effect.

½ cup cashew nut butter (see page 80)
⅛ cup maple syrup
⅛ cup agave
1 teaspoon Siberian ginseng
½ tablespoon astragalus
½ tablespoon taheebo
1 tablespoon foti
3 cups ice
¼ cup cacao powder
1 cup (250 mL) water

Place the nut butter, maple, and agave in a power blender. Add the herbs, ice, cacao powder, and water. Blend. You should get a thick, icy-textured drink that you can eat with a spoon. Sprinkle with cacao nibs.

When combining cacao and foti, an incredible synergy occurs. They support each other in effecting a powerful mood change by allowing greater levels of good-mood brain chemicals to become available.

Hot Beverages

When warming water for your hot beverages, don't boil the kettle as this will denature your water. Instead, parboil your water by turning the kettle off just as it starts to make a hissing noise.

Lexi's Cuppa Chai

This is the perfect warming drink on a cold winter's day.

4 cups (1 liter) water
4 cardamom pods
5 whole black peppercorns
1 nutmeg, whole
6 cloves, whole
6 allspice, whole
½ cinnamon stick, broken up
1 inch (2 cm) piece ginger, thinly sliced
1 deseeded vanilla pod, left over after using the seeds in one of the dessert recipes
2 rooibos tea bags
Pinch of cayenne pepper (optional, if you like it really spicy)
Pinch of buchu or mint (optional, if you want it minty)

2 cups (500 mL) Brazil nut milk
1 teaspoon ground cinnamon (optional)
1 tablespoon cacao powder (optional)

Place the water and spices in a pot on the stovetop over a low heat for approximately 1 hour to allow the spices to infuse the water. Make a batch of Brazil nut milk (see page 79). Strain the water from the spices, keeping the spices to reuse for a second steeping. Combine the Brazil nut milk and spiced water in a blender. Add cinnamon and cacao powder if desired. Serve immediately while still warm.

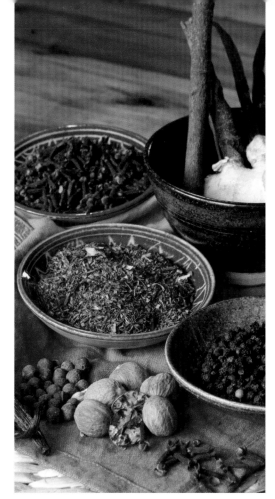
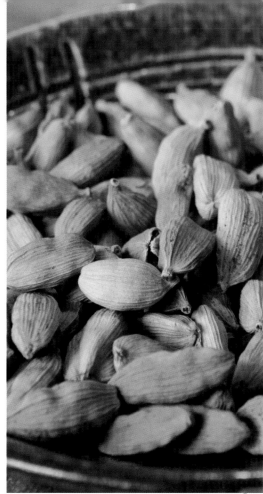

Mint-coca-sesame Tea

1½ cups (375 mL) hot water
1 cup (250 mL) sesame milk (see page 79)
3 coca tea bags, opened and the leaves emptied
1 tablespoon honey
1 inch (2 cm) chunk cacao butter
1 dried fig
1 drop of mint essential oil or 1 sprig of fresh mint

Blend all the ingredients in a power blender, pour into a cup, and drink immediately.

Coca tea is an invigorating herb made from the Andes Mountains' Coca plant. It is mainly used to increase the physical energy levels of the body.

Coff-tea

This is a tea mix that has the stimulating effect of coffee but gives you a gentle, energizing lift and no downer.

2 cups (500 mL) hot water
1 tablespoon green tea leaves
1 tablespoon yerba maté tea leaves
1 tablespoon coca tea leaves
1 tablespoon goji berries

Blend all the above ingredients and then sieve the brew.

1 tablespoon cacao powder
1 inch (2 cm) chunk cacao butter
1 tablespoon cashew nuts
Add honey to taste

Add the above ingredients to the tea base and blend again.

Yerba maté is an herbal tea that originate from South America. Th caffeine containing leaf used as a gentle stimula Traditionally, yerba ma is also used for treatmer of arthritis, slow digestic liver diseases, headache rheumatism, and obesit among others.

Hot Chocolate

1½ cups (375 mL) hot water
1 cup (250 mL) Brazil nut milk (see page 79)
2 tablespoons cacao powder, heaped
2 tablespoons cacao nibs
1 tablespoon honey
1 inch (2 cm) chunk cacao butter

Blend all the ingredients in a power blender, pour into a mug, and drink straight away.

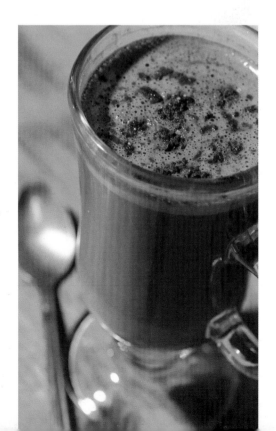

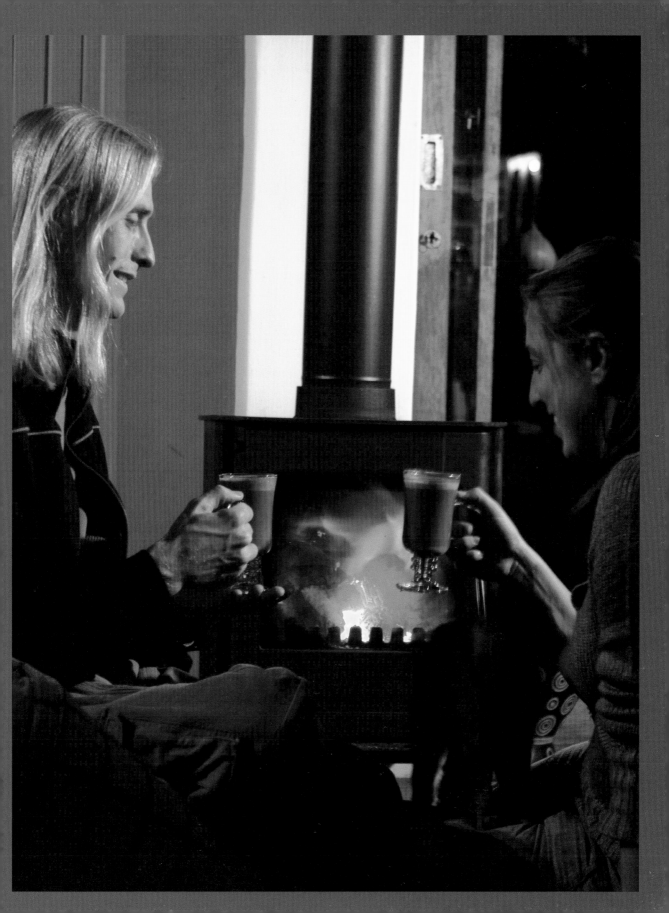

Recommended Reading

Information

The Sunfood Diet Success System, *David Wolfe*
Superfoods, *David Wolfe*
Conscious Eating, *Gabriel Cousens*
Ph Miracle, *Robert Young*
Raw Family: A True Story of Awakening, *Victoria Boutenko*
China Study, *T. Colin Campbell, Thomas M. Campbell*
The Complete Book of Raw Food, *Lori Baird*
Enzyme Nutrition, *Edward Howell*
Fats That Heal, Fats That Kill, *Udo Erasmus*
Living Foods for Optimum Health, *Brian R. Clement*
Green for Life, *Victoria Boutenko*
Naked Chocolate, *David Wolfe*
Depression-free for life, *Gabriel Cousens*
There Is a Cure for Diabetes, *Gabriel Cousens*
Wheat grass: Nature's Finest Medicine, *Steve Meyerowitz*
The Sprouting Book, *Ann Wigmore*
The Biophile magazine

Recipes

Rainbow Green Live-Food Cuisine, *Gabriel Cousens*
Rawvolution-Gourmet Living Cuisine, *Matt Amsden*
Everyday Raw, *Matthew Kenney*
Evie's Kitchen, *Shazzie*
Living in the Raw Gourmet, *Rose Lee Calabro*
I Am Grateful, *Terces Engelhart*
Fresh, *Valya Boutenko, Sergei Boutenko*
Ani's Raw Food Kitchen, *Ani Phyo*
The Raw Gourmet, *Nomi Shannon*

Visit our website for a more complete listing (see resources & links page).

Resources

Superfoods Webshop

www.superfoods.co.za

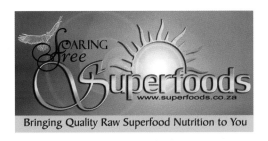

When we returned to South Africa we found that many of the superfoods that we were accustomed to eating were not available. We started importing our favorite superfoods mainly to keep ourselves and our friends in good supply. Very soon we were supplying the people on our workshops, then local health shops, specialized delis, and so on. We created our own brand dedicated to sourcing and distributing only the highest-quality organic superfoods we could find. We now have a wide and continuously growing range of superfoods available both in retail and bulk options.

Shop Online

We have a webshop that sells direct to the public. Over and above our own superfoods brand we have sourced other superfoods, super-supplements, and raw food items from local suppliers that support ongoing health. We only stock products that we are happy to use ourselves. Most American or European raw food books use ingredients that we cannot get hold of in South Africa. Every ingredient that we refer to in this book is either readily or seasonally available in your local fresh produce market, healthstore, or via our webshop. If you can't find something, get in touch and we will most likely be able to source it for you.

Visit our Office - Shop - Showroom

Our Soaring Free Superfoods headquarters are located in Cape Town. Please feel free to pop in, browse, shop, connect, and chat. We stock a full range of superfoods, wholefood supplements, kitchen equipment, and accessories, as well as raw food snacks and treats. Call 0861 000 976 or visit our website for directions.

Events

We travel around Southern Africa presenting the following events:

- Two-Day Raw Food Courses
- Chocolate Evenings
- Food Prep Classes
- Gourmet Retreats and Detox Juice Fasting Retreats

The two-day Raw Food Course is an introduction to the raw and living-foods lifestyle. Join us for two fun-filled days of essential know-how for healthy living and raw food preparation.

- *Reclaim your health (if it has gone missing).*
- *Lose weight and keep it off.*
- *Have abundant energy.*
- *Enhance your mental focus.*
- *Increase your vibration and awareness through the foods you choose.*

It's time to invest in yourself and your health. Learn how to uncook your food so that it tastes better than when it was cooked and is filled with living goodness.

Please visit the *Courses and Workshops* page at www.superfoods.co.za for more information on each of the various courses, workshops, retreats, and other events we are running. You will also find a current schedule of events on the website.

Feedback from past course participants:

"Lost 5 kilos (11 lbs) in 4 weeks – not dieting!!! Just healthy eating – Juicing is *amazing*."

"Invaluable info. Clarity on so many myths relating to food and *stunning* breakfast smoothies! I am wheat intolerant and have gained very useful info and recipes to help me."

"In a word: Wow! Positive, motivational. We have been armed with knowledge and support to make a raw lifestyle practical. I did not know that raw food could be sooo delicious!"

For more information or to book, please email info@superfoods.co.za or call 0861 000 976

Equipment

Our equipment of choice
When it comes to choosing a juicer, blender, dehydrator, or food processor there are many to choose from across a broad price range.

Choosing the best and the most practical
There's nothing worse than buying an expensive piece of kitchen equipment only to realize that if you'd spent just a little bit extra you would have had a better and more practical machine.

Juicer
The Oscar: This is a single-gear masticating juicer, meaning that it grinds your fruit or veg up slowly against a juicing screen instead of spinning it like a centrifugal juicer would do. This means that you get more of the goodness out of the produce. It juices all fruits and vegetables including green leafy veg and wheatgrass. It comes with a handy crushing screen, and is quiet and easy to clean.

Blender
The Vitamix: This is a high-speed power blender that will change your life.
You can put wet and dry ingredients into the jug and blend, grind, powder, pulverize, chop, mince, puree, or crush various ingredients.

Dehydrator
The Ezi Dri Ultra or Snackmaker: A dehydrator is a glorified hairdryer. It has a fan at the bottom that blows and circulates warm air through the trays. The two brands mentioned here are dehydrators that allow you to set the drying temperature to your desired setting. Remember it is important to warm or dry your food at low temperatures so as not to destroy the enzymes, nutrients, and vitamins. There is no point buying a cheap dehydrator that only has one drying setting of over 158°F (70°C).

Food Processor
The Magimix: This food processor is the top-of-the-range sturdy, all-purpose chopping and mixing appliance. It comes with useful grating and slicing attachments.

All of the above-mentioned equipment comes with reliable guarantees, servicing options, and replaceable parts.

Call our office on 0861 000 976 or Healthmakers on 0861 100 695 for orders or enquiries.

Raw Food Resources: A Select American and UK List

The raw food movement has been growing by leaps and bounds in recent years. This is just a starting point for your explorations, to stock a few of the most important kitchen basics and discover some of the terrific raw food restaurants out there.

United States

RAW KITCHEN EQUIPMENT

Vitamix Power Blender
8615 Usher Road
Cleveland, OH 44138-2199
Phone: 800-848-2649
www.vitamix.com

Oscar Juicer
On the World Wide Web
6366 Commerce Blvd #200
Rohnert Park, CA 94928
www.discountjuicers.com

Nature's First Law
P.O. Box 900202
San Diego, CA 92190
Phone: 800-205-2350
www.rawfood.com

RAW RESTAURANTS

For a more complete listing of raw food restaurants in the U.S. and beyond, please visit www.soystache.com/raw-food-restaurants.htm.

Tree of Life Café
P.O. Box 1080
Patagonia, AZ 85624
www.treeoflife.nu
Café Gratitude

1730 Shattuck Ave
Berkeley, CA 94709
415-824-4652
www.cafegratitude.com

118 Degrees
2981 Bristol St., Suite B-5
Costa Mesa, CA 92626
714-754-0718
www.shop118degrees.com/index.html

Cru Cafe
1521 Griffith Park Blvd.
Los Angeles, CA 90026
323-667-1551
http://crusilverlake.com/

Raw Life Foods Cafe
"If you eat alive, you stay alive!"
1714 West 3rd Street
Montgomery, AL 36106-1506
334-834-4425

Mooi
1700 W Sunset Blvd
Los Angeles, CA 90026
213-413-1100

RAW-FOOD INSTRUCTION, LIFESTYLE TRAINING, AND RETREATS

The Tree of Life Rejuvenation Center
P.O. Box 1080
Patagonia, AZ 85624
Phone: 520-394-2520
E-mail: healing@treeoflife.nu

David Wolfe's Longevity Website:
www.bestdayever.com

Hippocrates Health Institute
1443 Palmdale Court
West Palm Beach, FL 33411
Phone: 800-842-2125
www.hippocratesinst.com

Living Light Culinary Arts Institute
Cherie Soria, Director
704 N. Harrison
Fort Bragg, CA 95437
Phone: 800-6933 ext. 6256

Victoria, Sergei, and Valya Boutenko's Raw Family site
www.rawfamily.com

United Kingdom

RAW KITCHEN EQUIPMENT

Vitamix Power Blender
Vitamix Europe Ltd.
The Old Library
6 Linden Rd.
Clevedon, North Somerset
BS21 7SN
United Kingdom
Phone: UK Local Rate:
08458684566
IE Local Rate: 0766709854
Other: +1 440 235 4840

Oscar Juicer
www.vitality4life.co.uk

Magimix Food Processor
enquiries@magimix-spares.co.uk
Telephone: 01252 727755 (UK)
+44 1252 727755 (outside UK)
Fax: 01252 727766 (UK)
+44 1252 727766 (outside UK)
BBS Ltd
Unit B
Grovebell Industrial Estate
Wrecclesham Road
Farnham, Surrey GU10 4PL
England

RAW RESTAURANTS

Manna
Manna is a pioneering organic Live/Powerfood cafe and musical oasis. www.galaxyofvitality.com/manna
24 Coombe Rd
Brighton
East Sussex, London BN2 4EA
01273 690 540

Dragonfly Wholefoods
Raw Food Café & Raw Home Delivery Service
http://dragonflywholefoods.co.uk/bistro.html
24 Highgate High Street
Highgate, London N6 5JG
tel. 0208 347 6087

Saf Restauant
(Chef Chad Sarno)
www.safrestaurant.co.uk
152-154 Curtain Road
Shoreditch, London EC2A 3AT
+44 (0)20 76130 007

Vita Organic
www.vitaorganic.co.uk
74 Wardour Street
London, England W1F 0TE
0207 734 8986

Alchemy THC SuperLifeFood
Pure Vegetarian Deli & Store
1 Omega Place Kings Cross
London, England
+44(0)7917446455/78375223

Amitay Point
(raw-friendly restaurant)
www.amitypoint.co.uk
16 Onley St., Norwich. UK. NR2 2EB

RAW-FOOD INSTRUCTION, LIFESTYLE TRAINING, AND RETREATS

www.totalrawfood.com
www.shazzie.com
ww.rawliving.com

Peter Pure
www.rawfoodparty.com
Phone: 01733 759648

Raw Food Forum

We have created a raw food forum on our website, www.superfoods.co.za.

Once you have registered you will be able to chat with other raw food enthusiasts, exchange ideas and recipes, and ask questions. There are further resource sections on the forum as well as on the resources & links page of the website, where you will find details of local fresh produce suppliers, well-stocked health shops, delis, raw-friendly restaurants, excellent workshops on growing your own food, and other interesting and related sites.

There is a fast-growing community of raw, health-conscious people in Southern Africa. Although at first a change of lifestyle such as the one described in this book can seem extreme and isolating, when we scratch the surface just a little bit we find rich and fertile soil; like-minded people who are embracing change, willing to connect, and wanting to create supportive and sustainable communities that touch and tread lightly on the Earth.

To your health, joy, and freedom.

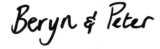

Contact details

www.superfoods.co.za

Office hours:
9am – 4pm
Tel: 0861 000976
International tel: +27 21 683 5008
Fax: 086 668 2777

Email:
info@superfoods.co.za

Postal address:
PostNet Suite 354, Private bag X16
Constantia, 7848
Cape Town, South Africa

Index